Dr. Me

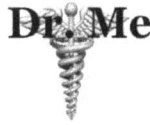

Patient & Caregiver Self-Help Guide

Dr.Me, LLC
9249 S. Broadway, #200-408
Highlands Ranch, CO. 80129

Ordering Information:
Quantity sales: Discounts are available on quantity purchases. For details contact the publisher at the address above. Orders by U.S. trade bookstores and wholesalers. Please contact Dr.Me: (303) 809-5760.

Printed in the United States of America.
First Printing, 2018
ISBN: 978-0-9985708-0-8

Introduction

Health care in the United States is a big and complicated business. It is funded by and delivered through a combination of powerful public and private organizations. All of them have interests that conflict with the best interests of patients.

Today, the business of medicine makes it difficult for even the best doctors to find the time and the resources to help their patients solve their health care problems. These same doctors, as well as nurses and hospital executives, struggle themselves to get safe, quality health care when they become patients.

This *Patient and Caregiver Guide* was developed to help you control your health care choices and finances any time that you engage with our complicated and broken health care system.

The *Guide* walks you step by step through solutions to almost any health care access, quality, or financial situation. Throughout these pages, you'll find contacts, phone numbers, education, tips, guidance, information, and connections to experts and resources that can help you get the safest, highest-quality, and most cost-efficient health care possible.

Regardless of your age, income, or circumstances your health and well-being are likely among the most important aspects of your life. Yet, when it comes to our health, we often place our trust blindly in physicians who have limited time to guide us, in hospitals that we know little about, and in a health care system that kills and injures millions of people every year due to safety, quality, and cost issues.

Tip: Counting on doctors and other health care professionals to ensure that you get the safest, highest-quality, and most affordable health care increases your risk of becoming a victim.

You can dramatically influence your own health outcomes and well-being through your choices about your diet, activity, self-care, insurance, doctors, treatments, finances, and engagement with your health care teams.

The bottom line is that you must take an active role in your own health care to ensure the best outcomes. The best way to accomplish this is through three simple rules that every person can follow:

1. Ask questions until you fully understand your circumstances and choices.
2. Make sure that your preferences are heard.
3. Follow through until your concerns are addressed.

Unfortunately, our broken, fragmented, and complicated health care system makes it difficult for patients and their caregivers to collaborate with their health care providers.

So, how do you overcome these obstacles?

- Become and stay fully engaged with your health, doctors, and health care teams.
- Learn everything you can about your condition and circumstances when you are diagnosed with an illness.

- Know your health insurance.
- Get qualified and expert help whenever needed.

To help you meet any health care challenge, every section of the *Guide* provides:

Step-by-step instructions
Explanations
Tips
Experts and resources
Phone numbers
Websites
Contact information
Education

To ensure that you can easily access updated and comprehensive information, the *Dr.Me Guide*, provides a companion Mobile Help Index, available 24/7, at www.aPatientsPlace.com.

Control Your Health

The top health risk factors haven't changed much over the years. They include smoking, being overweight, having a bad diet, not getting enough exercise, maintaining high levels of ongoing stress, high blood pressure, and high cholesterol.

Your choices have an immediate impact on these risk factors. Your income, race, gender, and circumstances are not major factors.

The keys to reducing your health risks are to identify which ones pertain to you, understand them, and start taking little positive steps that are easy for you to add to your life every day. Some examples include:

- Substituting one glass of water for one glass of soda each day.
- Taking a walk around your block once a day when you would normally sit and watch TV.
- Replacing one high-fat, high-sugar meal with a salad.
- Getting a free blood pressure test and/or health screening each year.
- Screening and choosing a doctor to serve as your primary care physician.

Tip: Trying to make major changes quickly is not usually effective or long-lasting.

The best ways to take control of your health care are to:

1. Stay as healthy as possible by taking good care of yourself.
2. Use as many free and low-cost screenings as possible.
3. Keep your health care costs down.
4. Work with your doctors and health care teams.
5. Strengthen the areas of your body that are weak.

Pay attention to your body's natural signals that something may be wrong. You can't control your genetics, but you can control what you do about your individual risk factors.

The Earlier the Better

Another way to take control of your health care is to recognize potential problems early, learn what to do when you spot a problem, and discuss with your doctor what's treatable by yourself and what needs medical attention.

Once you know how to spot common health problems early and what to do when you find them, you can stop minor and routine issues from becoming complicated and costly health problems.

Tip: More than 80% of all health problems are cared for in the home.

Since each person's actions and choices have a major impact on their health and well-being, patients must be at the center of their own health care teams to get safe, quality health care.

Fortunately, there are many tools to help us today, and many others are in development. Online symptom checkers, free helplines, wearable devices, virtual doctor appointments, home-health monitoring, insurance provider portals, online patient communities, free medical bill review services, and others are a few of the resources available to help patients manage their health care and engage with their doctors and health care team members.

Today, more than 20% of physicians are using mobile technology with their patients, and a 2015 survey of 500 doctors by the Texas firm Research Now concluded that almost half of the physicians surveyed planned to adopt mobile apps to communicate with their patients.[1] Related research found that 96% of consumers using mobile health care apps believed that their devices are helping them improve the quality of their lives.[2] Calorie counters, blood pressure monitoring, and activity tracking are among the most popular apps, and new apps are being developed almost daily.

One example of how mobile health care applications are helping patients with chronic illnesses is a project by Banner Health called Intensive Ambulatory Care. This project uses multiple mobile devices for home health monitoring to help 600 patients with multiple chronic conditions. Results from the initial 135-patient pilot program showed a 27% reduction in the costs of care.[3] This was primarily due to a decrease in hospital admissions, shorter lengths of stay, and lower outpatient costs.[4]

The program demonstrated the commonly held thought that mobile devices can have many beneficial results when they are used in a structured system. Conversely, the same mobile devices can increase risks due to a lack of care coordination and misleading information when they used in a nonstructured environment.[5]

Tip: Review and contribute to an updated and categorized list of leading health care apps by using your smartphone or laptop to access www.aPatientsPlace.com.

Even though the best medicine is staying healthy, this *Guide* does not discuss all that goes into keeping physically, emotionally, and spiritually healthy. Maintaining your health and wellness deserves its own focus. Instead, this *Guide* focuses on ensuring that you can take control and optimize your health care whenever you suspect that something may be wrong with your health.

Tip: Only you can optimize your health and well-being.

Let's look at some of the basic steps required to take control of your health care, work with your physicians and health insurance provider, and manage your health care–related finances.

Step 1: Control Your Choices

Unless you experience a medical emergency and you are not conscious, you can control your health care choices. You are the master of your body and life. While you can't choose when you get a serious injury or illness, in all nonemergency situations, you do get to choose what to do about them.

To make good choices, you'll likely need help from family, friends, health professionals, and other experts. The question is, how do you learn enough to make the right choices when your doctors have fifteen minutes on average for an appointment, your medical records from other doctors and providers may not be accessible by your health team when needed, and it's virtually impossible to tell exactly how much tests and treatments your physician recommends will cost?

Tip: Connecting to people who have already gone through a similar diagnosis is extremely helpful. Leading online patient communities are discussed in Section 3, and a complete and updated list can be found at www.aPatientsPlace.com.

Step 2: Ask Who, What, Where, When, Why, and How Much, All the Time

If you accept everything you are told by your health providers without asking questions, you are increasing your risk of being the victim of mistakes, getting lower quality health care, and spending more money than you need. If you don't ask questions, who do you think will? If you don't tell your doctors and health providers what you want, how will they know?

Researchers at the world-renowned Johns Hopkins Medicine estimate that more than 250,000 Americans die, and many more are injured, every year from medical errors.[6] The more common preventable errors are:

- Patients being misdiagnosed because doctors are hurrying and are reluctant to ask a second physician's opinion.
- Health care providers mixing up the names of drugs to be administered to patients.
- Hospital-acquired infections. This occurs in 5 to 10% of all patients admitted to acute care and long-term care facilities in the United States.
- Surgical errors—both reported and unreported. In many cases, the errors occur after surgery due to failure to diagnose common complications.

Data from the U.S. government estimates that as many as 80% of hospital bills contain mistakes.[7] If you don't ask about your out-of-pocket costs, negotiate fees when you can, and review all your bills for errors, you are increasing the risk that you will pay more than you need.

The prior examples only scratch the tip of the problem. The important thing to remember is that your actions can ensure that you are not victimized by the problems that have become a part of the health care system.

Step 3: Controlling Health Care Quality and Safety

The most important steps you can take to ensure that you get the safest and highest quality health care possible are to become a smart health care consumer and to be involved in decision making all the time.

Quality health care means different things to different people. Some people think that getting quality health care is seeing the doctor right away whenever they want. Other people feel that quality health care is being treated courteously by the doctor's staff and having a doctor spend a lot of time with them. Still others think quality health care means that their insurance provider does not put them on hold for ten minutes every time they call to get answers to basic questions.

According to the National Committee for Quality Assurance (NCQA) quality health care is:

- Doing the right thing (getting the health care services you need),
- at the right time (when you need them),
- in the right way (using the appropriate test or procedure),
- to achieve the best possible results.[8]

Whatever your definition of "quality" is, what matters most is:

- Ensuring that you get the safest and highest quality health care possible.
- Getting a quick and accurate diagnosis.
- Finding the most effective treatment and/or management for your condition or illness.
- Making sure that your treatment and care is coordinated between everyone on your health care team(s).
- Recovering and returning to the highest quality of life possible given your situation.
- Managing your health care finances so you do not pay more than you need to.

You might think that every doctor, nurse, pharmacist, and hospital provides high-quality care. Unfortunately, this is not the case. As noted earlier, doctors, hospitals, pharmacists, therapists, drug providers, equipment manufacturers, and suppliers all serve other interests than the patient's. Some of these health care providers struggle financially. They all have trade groups and industry organizations lobbying for their interests.

The quality of health care services delivered to each patient varies depending on where you live, what providers you see, when you see your providers, how much experience your providers have in diagnosing and treating your condition, and other factors. Quality also varies from state to state and from one doctor's office to another.

Tips for controlling costs:

- *You pay less when you use in-network providers.*

- *Take advantage of free tests and preventive screenings held in your area.*
- *Use urgent care centers instead of emergency rooms unless you have a true emergency.*
- *Ask your doctor or pharmacist about generic versus brand-name drugs.*
- *Organize and keep track of your medical records.*
- *Follow through on your doctor's prescribed treatments*

Step 4: Plan for the Worst—Advance Directives

Advance directives are written instructions that allow you to state what you'd prefer if you are too ill to make your wishes known. Your family and doctors will follow your advance directives if you are unable to make your own health care decisions. Anyone age 18 or older may prepare advance directives.

Tip: Each state has its own laws regarding advance directives.

There are three main kinds of advance directives: living wills, health care proxies, and Do Not Resuscitate (DNR) orders.

A **living will** is a written, legal document that spells out the types of medical treatments and life-sustaining measures you do and don't want. These often include mechanical breathing (respiration and ventilation), tube feeding, or resuscitation. In some states, living wills may be called health care declarations or health care directives.

A **health care proxy** is more detailed than a living will. It allows you to appoint the person or persons you trust to make health decisions for you if you cannot. It also allows for more detailed advance care planning such as your wishes about resuscitation, feeding tubes, antibiotics, hospital transfers, respirators, and more. Because the health care proxy involves more decisions, you may want to talk to your doctor about various options for care. For instance, many people would be willing to try a feeding tube or a ventilator for a while, but then want it to be stopped if their condition did not improve.

Also, talk to family members and the person(s) you have appointed as your proxy to be sure they understand your wishes. A health care proxy is also known as a medical or health care power of attorney, sometimes referred to as a MPOA or a HCPOA.

A **Do Not Resuscitate (DNR)** order is a request not to have cardiopulmonary resuscitation (CPR) if your heart stops or if you stop breathing. Advance directives do not have to include a DNR order, and you don't have to have an advance directive to have a DNR order. Your doctor can put a DNR order in your medical chart.

Advance care directives are legally valid everywhere in the United States, but laws concerning them vary from state to state. Forms approved for the state you live in are available from many different health care organizations and institutions.

Unexpected end-of-life situations can happen at any age. All adults should have advance directives. Injury, illness, and death aren't easy subjects to talk about. With careful planning, you can ensure that you receive the type of medical care you want, and that you have taken the burden off your family and loved ones for trying to guess what you would have wanted.

Discussing Advance Directives

Follow these steps to get the conversation going about your wishes in the event you are unable to speak for yourself.

Step 1: Start the Conversation

Let your loved ones know that you want to implement advance directives. There are many great online resources that provide suggestions on how to start the dialogue with your family.

Step 2: Explain Your Feelings

It's generally best to approach the subject in a matter-of-fact and reassuring manner. However, make sure you get your feelings across about medical care and what you'd want done in specific instances. Keep in mind that a living will cannot cover every possible situation. Therefore, you may also want a medical power of attorney (MPOA) to designate someone to be your health care agent.

An MPOA will be guided by your living will, but he or she will have the authority to interpret your wishes in situations that aren't described in your living will. An

MPOA may also be a good idea if your family is opposed to some of your wishes or they are divided about them.

Step 3: Choose a Health Care Agent

Choosing a person to act as your health care agent may be the most important part of your planning. You need to trust that this person will have your best interests at heart, understand your wishes, and will act accordingly. She or he should also be mature, level-headed, and comfortable with candid conversations. Don't pick someone out of feelings of guilt or obligation.

Your health care agent does not need to be a family member. You may want your health care decision agent to be different from the person you choose to handle your financial matters. It is easier, but not necessary, if the person you choose lives in the same city or state as you do.

Step 4: Identify the Treatments You Want

Think about what's important to you. For example, is it important to remain independent and self-sufficient, or what would make your life not worth living? Would you want treatment to extend your life in any situation? Would you want treatment only if a cure is possible? Would you want palliative care to ease pain and discomfort if you were terminally ill? Although you can't predict what medical situations will arise, be sure to discuss the following treatments:

Resuscitation. Restarts the heart when it has stopped

beating (also known as cardiac death). Determine when you would want to be resuscitated by cardiopulmonary resuscitation (CPR) or by a device that delivers an electric shock to stimulate the heart.

Mechanical ventilation. Takes over your breathing if you're unable to breathe on your own. Consider if, when, and for how long you would want to be placed on a mechanical ventilator.

Nutritional and hydration assistance. Supplies the body with nutrients and fluids intravenously, or via a tube in the stomach. Decide if, when, and for how long you would want to be fed in this manner.

Dialysis. Removes waste from your blood and manages fluid levels if your kidneys no longer function. Determine if, when, and for how long you would want to receive this treatment.

You can also specify in your advance directives any wishes about donating your organs, eyes, and tissue for transplantation or your body for scientific study.

Tip: If you wish to donate your body for scientific study, contact the medical school closest to your home for details.

Your advance directives should be in writing. Fill out the forms for your state. Although it isn't required, you may want to consult an attorney about this process. State-specific forms are available from a variety of websites. The National Hospice and Palliative Care Organization has the forms for most states available on its website (www.nhpco.org).

Once you've filled out the forms, give copies to your doctor, the person you've chosen as your health care agent, and your family members. Your instinct might be to put your advance directives somewhere safe, like a safe-deposit box, but that will only make it difficult for your loved ones to find the forms when they need them.

Review your advance directives from time to time. As your health changes or your perspective on life changes, you might reconsider some of your advance directives. Also, consider if you want to revise any of the instructions. You can change your mind about your advance directives at any time.

To revise your advance directives, you follow the same steps you used to create them.

- Get new advance directive forms to fill out.
- Discuss your changes with your friends, family, and doctor.
- Distribute copies of the new advance directives and ask everyone to destroy the earlier version.

Tip: If there isn't time to redo the paperwork, you can always cancel your advance directive by telling your doctor and your family.

Remember, a living will or MPOA only goes into effect if you are unable to make medical decisions for yourself, as determined by your doctors.

Controlling your choices, asking questions, and advanced planning will help ensure that you get safe and quality health care. No doubt, some day you will find yourself needing the help of a doctor or other health provider. This *Guide* is for that day. However, it is just a guide; there are other resources you can use in conjunction with it.

Find a trusted friend or loved one to help you. If you do not have anyone in your life who you feel can help you, ask your doctor for resources in your community that are available. If your doctor does not help, call the patient services department at your local hospital. If that does not work, go to the library and search the Internet for help in your local area. Every community has help. You do not need to be alone.

This rest of this *Guide* will take you through each step to safe, quality, and affordable health care. Leading your health teams starts by making health a priority and listening to your body. When you suspect something might be wrong, use this *Guide* and Dr. Me's mobile help index at www.aPatientsPlace.com to get all of the help you need.

However, if you choose to simply let things happen, do as you're told by your health care and insurance providers, not question anything, or advocate for yourself, then you are choosing to accept the possibility of riskier, lower quality, and more expensive health care. The choice is yours.

SECTION 1
You Must Fight for Yourself

As a patient in the U.S. health care system you will face many obstacles to getting safe, quality, and affordable health care. To overcome them, you must advocate for yourself and lead your health care team. You'll get a big assist from many primary and specialty care practices transitioning into medical homes and providing patient-centered care.

You are the core of your health. You make the most of the choices that impact your health. You certainly feel or suspect that something may be wrong long before anyone else. You decide when and how to engage with the health care system.

The crucial steps when advocating for yourself are:

- Ask questions when you're not sure.
- Get your questions answered in a way that you understand
- Make sure that your preferences are known by your health care providers and caregivers.

Four reasons you must advocate for yourself, and lead your health care teams are:

1. You'll improve the safety, quality, and affordability of your health care by taking responsibility for and control of your health care choices. Frankly, that should be more

than enough reason to communicate and work with your doctors and other health care team members.

2: There is no guaranteed that anyone else will advocate for you, especially when things get difficult. Your primary care physician (PCP) might try. However, it is a rare exception when a PCP or his or her staff has time to advocate for their patients for anything but the most basic issues and finances. Even if your PCP is fantastic about helping you understand your choices and advocating on your behalf, no one knows your body, health, and preferences better than you.

Even if you're fortunate enough to have family members or loved ones to make sure that your interests are heard and protected, there are limits to how much they can help. It's critical for you to remain engaged and involved, guiding and communicating with your health care teams and providers.

3: Every health care professional or provider you interact with, including your doctor(s), has other interests to consider. Doctors serve many patients, their staff, their investors, the needs of their practice, and sometimes their own self-interests. Hospital case managers, discharge planners, and service representatives at your health insurance company, Medicare, and Medicaid can help you with your policy, coverage, care coordination, and choices. However, they, too, have other professional and financial interests that are not necessarily aligned with your interests.

Tip: Decisions about your benefits are all too often influenced by your health insurers' ability to control costs or make money.

4: Advocating for yourself empowers you. Positive

emotions like empowerment are good for our physical and emotional well-being, including helping to speed recovery time. Advocating for yourself also helps to lower the risk of medical mistakes, and it often reduces the cost of health care.

Everyone can advocate for themselves. You just need to know how.

Tip: Seniors and people with language barriers tend to be the most passive in the doctor-patient relationship. If you are an older patient or have challenges understanding English, consider having another person go with you to appointments.

Advocating for Yourself Can Be Tough

Speaking up for yourself can be difficult and even scary at times. It is especially difficult when you are just starting to advocate for yourself and you are speaking with doctors and other health professionals who have a lot of education and experience.

You can make it easier to have those conversations by following these six steps:

Step 1: Listen to and Understand Your Own Body

You don't need to worry that the doctor will know more than you. Nobody knows *you* better than you. See Section 3 in this *Guide* for more information.

Step 2: Get Copies of Your Past Records

Take the time to understand your medical records. If you're not 100% certain what things mean, contact the treating physician's office and ask for an explanation. Sharing this information is another good way to begin a dialogue with your doctor.

Step 3: Learn as Much as Possible about Your Family's Health History

Telling your doctor about your family history will help him or her understand any potential genetic issues.

Step 4: Learn Everything Possible about Your Condition and Your Insurance Coverage

Learning about your condition and insurance coverage will make you a much better advocate for yourself. There is much more information in this *Guide* about researching your condition or illness and learning about your health insurance.

Step 5: Consider Your Needs and Preferences

Your needs and preferences include learning what your rights are and where you can get assistance, support, and trustworthy information. There is more information later in the *Guide*.

Tip: An ideal patient-doctor relationship optimizes the

medical expertise of the doctor with the situational knowledge and preferences of the patient.

Step 6: Your Goals in Self-Advocating

Your goals in self-advocating are to fully understand your circumstances and choices, and to make your voice and preferences heard. It does not matter whether you are speaking using sign language, or using assistive technology. Effective communication is not angry or demanding. It is respectful and understanding, even though the answers at times may be frustrating.

Tip: You are the person with the most at stake. So you need to have control over what happens to the best of your ability.

You Are the Boss of You

You have the right to respectful and considerate treatment from all doctors and health care providers. Expect and demand nothing less. You choose your doctor(s). You can and should replace them if needed. You can refuse any test or treatment without giving an explanation. Unless you are on Medicaid, Medicare, or public assistance, you also choose your insurance.

Speaking Up at a Hospital or a Nursing Home

If you have a concern while you're in the hospital, you should immediately tell someone who is directly involved with your care.

Tip: If you are not 100% sure why you are being given a drug or you are told that a test has been scheduled, ask for more information before agreeing to move forward. Your first option should be your doctor, then a nurse, then a floor or unit manager.

Providers need your help in resolving problems quickly before they become bigger problems. When you tell someone about your concerns, also tell them what you want and what you expect them to do about it.

Tip: If you do not receive a timely response, consider contacting the hospital customer service, patient advocacy, or patient safety/quality department

Be Prepared

The world-renowned Johns Hopkins Medicine (JHM) suggests that you prepare a kit with important medical information before you go into any hospital or treatment facility. Your kit should include your medical information, including medications and dosages, any allergies, names and contact information of your physicians, your insurance company, and a designated person to speak for you if you are unable to speak for yourself.

JHM also suggests that you:

- Bring someone to help or advocate for you.

- Always asks question, especially regarding medications, tests, procedures, and doctors that are scheduled to see you.
- Start and keep moving as quickly as possible, consistent with your doctor's instructions.
- Help prevent infections by asking anyone who visits to wash their hands or use hand sanitizer.
- Discuss your discharge and care coordination plans when you are getting ready for release from the hospital or facility.

Tip: A copy of your discharge summary should be given to you and your primary care physician when you are discharged. If it's not, make sure you get a copy soon after you are discharged.

Consumer Reports has published an excellent hospital survival guide to help you get the highest quality care while you are in a treatment facility. Their guide includes checklists to remind you what to do starting with "before you are admitted," continuing through to "when you check in," "during your stay," and "when you leave." The guide can be found online at http://www.consumerreports.org/cro/2012/10/your-hospital-survival-guide/index.htm.

Your Advocacy Skills

Once you start paying attention to your body and you understand that you can control your health care choices and finances, you can start working on the critical skills you'll need to advocate for yourself.

These must-have skills are quite simple. They start with asking questions and telling people what you need. Other skills that are very helpful include:

Skill 1: Understanding Your Health Insurance

Many people don't understand the basics of their health insurance. You can take the following steps to fix this:

- Write down your questions regarding your insurance.
- Call your insurance customer service.
- Request a copy of your policy.
- Explain your circumstances.
- Ask as many questions as needed until you understand your benefits, coverage, and expected costs.

Before you hang up with your health insurance customer service representative, ask who you can call if you have more questions and how familiar that person will be with your circumstances.

If you don't have health insurance, or you use Medicaid, Medicare, or public assistance, contact your state health department for details about your coverage, or use www.benefitscheckup.org to find free programs and services in your area that can help you get the information you need.

Skill 2: Researching and Gathering Information

A key component of self-advocacy and good decision making is learning as much as possible about your illness and circumstances.

Your doctors, other patients, Internet health portals, professional medical associations, your health insurance provider, and other health professionals are all valid sources of information. Consult Sections 3 and 10 in this *Guide* for step-by-step instructions on learning about your condition.

Tip: No single health care professional has all the answers for you

Skill 3: Communication

The people involved with your health care must understand your needs, concerns, and questions if they are going to help you. The most important steps in communicating effectively are to ask questions, listen carefully to the responses, and make sure that you express your needs until you can confirm that you have been heard.

Skill 4: Problem Solving

There are many decisions that you may need to make throughout your diagnosis, treatment, and recovery. Examples include whether to get a second opinion, have a specific test or treatment, find a new doctor, choose a hospital, participate in a clinical trial, and much more.

Skill 5: Negotiating

At numerous times, you may find yourself having to persuade others to get what you want. It may be as simple as leaving the hospital a day early, or more complicated like obtaining a different prescription or negotiating a discount for services. When you find yourself having to argue for what you want, your negotiating skills may be put to the test.

Skill 6: Preparation

Another self-advocacy skill that is not often mentioned is preparation. When you are prepared, you save everyone time, and you can contribute more to your health care teams. To prepare, do your research, keep records, think about your preferences, suggest solutions, keep an open mind, and work in partnership with others to solve problems. Remember, you are not alone.

Tip: A great way to learn what to expect is to speak with other patients and caregivers who have already experienced what you are just beginning to go through. There are many patient-to-patient communities (online and in person) that you can access for free. Links to several leading patient communities are included throughout this Guide *and online at* www.aPatientsPlace.com.

Skill 7: Writing a Complaint Letter

When a problem is not resolved to your satisfaction through phone calls or face-to-face conversation, you can write a letter and send it directly to the hospital or the facility where you were treated. You can even file a formal complaint with your state regulatory agency.

Include the following in a complaint letter:

- Your name, address, and phone number.
- The date(s) of your treatment.
- The name(s) of the health care provider(s) who cared for you.
- A short overview of your complaint.
- A statement about what you would like to see happen next.
- Copies of any supporting document or attachments (keep the originals).

Tip: Consider sending copies to others who can help solve the problem. Also, keep the originals organized in a safe place that you will remember.

Find Free Help Fast

Tip: If you need help advocating for yourself or a loved one, contact the Patient Advocate Foundation by phone at 800-532-5274. Their service is free, and they have professional case managers to help you. They have helped hundreds of thousands of families since 1996. You can learn more about them online at www.patientadvocate.org/.

Free Helplines for Specific Diseases and Illnesses

Find additional and updated phone numbers and resources at www.aPatientsPlace.com.

Alzheimer's 24/7 Helpline: 800-272-3900
American Breast Cancer Foundation: 410-730-5105
American Cancer Society: 800-227-2345
American Childhood Cancer Organization: 855-858-2226
American Institute for Cancer Research: 800-843-8114
American Kidney Fund: 866-300-2900
The Assistance Fund: 855-845-3663
BenefitsCheckUp: 571-527-3900
Blood & Marrow Transplant Network: 888-597-7674
CancerCare: 800-813-4673
Cancer Hope Network: 800-552-4366
Caring Vice Coalition (chronic illnesses): 888-267-1440
Center for Medicare Advocacy: 860-456-7790; 202-293-5760
Chai Lifeline (childhood illnesses): 877-242-4543
Colon Cancer Alliance: 877-422-2030
National Center for Complementary and Alternative Medicine: 888-644-6226
Gilda Radner Familial Ovarian Cancer Registry: 800-682-7426
Good Days (chronic diseases): 877-968-7233
International Myeloma Foundation: 800-452-2873
Kidney Disease Helpline: 800-891-5390
Leukemia & Lymphoma Society: 800-955-4572
LIVESTRONG (cancer): 855-220-7777
Lung Cancer Alliance: 800-298-2436
Medicare Rights Center: 800-333-4114
Medication Assistance Helpline: 800-503-6897
National Alliance on Mental Illness: 800-950-6264

National Bone Marrow Transplant Link: 800-546-5268
National Cancer Institute: 800-422-6237
National Domestic Violence Hotline: 800-799-7233
National Eye Institute: 301-496-5248
National Kidney Foundation: 855-653-2273
National Organization for Rare Disorders: 203-744-0100
National Patient Travel Center: 800-296-1217
National Psoriasis Foundation: 800-723-9166
National Sexual Assault Hotline: 800-656-4673
National Stroke Association: 800-787-6537
National Suicide Prevention Hotline: 800-273-8255
Pancreatic Cancer Action Network: 877-272-6226
Patient Access Network Foundation: 866-316-7263
Patient Advocate Foundation: 800-532-5274
Patient Assistance Programs (prescription drugs): 877-267-0517
St. Jude's Hospital (childhood cancer): 866-278-5833
Substance Abuse and Mental Health Services
Administration: 800-662-4357
Susan G Komen (breast cancer): 212-560-9590
U.S Department of Health and Human Services (aging):
800-677-1116
Us TOO International (prostate cancer): 800-808-7866
Veterans Crisis Line: 888-457-4838

Patient Advocacy Organizations

Caregiver Action Network
http://caregiveraction.org/

Consumers Advancing Patient Safety

http://patientsafety.org/

Empowered Patient Coalition
http://empoweredpatientcoalition.org/

Hospice Patients Alliance
http://hospicepatients.org/

Medically Induced Trauma Support Services
http://www.mitss.org/

Patient Advocate Foundation
http://www.patientadvocate.org/

Patients with Disabilities

If you have a disability, you have a right to accessible health care under federal, state, and local laws. The most important of those laws is the Americans with Disabilities Act (ADA) and Section 504 of the Rehabilitation Act of 1973. ADA and Section 504 require medical providers to ensure that people with disabilities have access to equivalent services as other patients.

Under these laws, you are considered an individual with a disability if you have a physical or mental impairment that substantially limits a major life activity, have a record of an impairment, or have already been designated with such an impairment. Major life activities include but are not limited to: seeing, hearing, walking, working, and major bodily functions. For more information on your rights as a disabled person, use the following links and resources.

American Foundation for the Blind
Disability rights resources for people with vision loss.
www.afb.org

Americans with Disabilities Act
www.ada.gov

Advocating Change Together
A grassroots disability rights organization run by and for people with disabilities.
www.selfadvocacy.org

A 2015 article written by Elizabeth Renter in *U.S. News and World Report* mentions the following six ways to become a better self-advocate:

1. Understand your health insurance, especially the basics of your coverage. A recent report from the Kaiser Family Foundation found the more than 40% of people don't understand basic health insurance terms, and many more were completely lost when asked to calculate how much they would have to pay out-of-pocket for specific hospitalizations.

2. Prepare to ask questions of your doctor(s) and health care providers. Make a list of your questions before your appointment. You may have very limited time to get the answers that you want, so be prepared.

3. Maintain your medical records. It can be a major hassle to get your medical records transferred from one provider to another. Ask for copies of your

records whenever you check in for an appointment. Step-by-step instructions are included in Section 16 of this *Guide.*

4. Review your medical bills for errors. An estimated 80% of medical medicals contain errors, the only way that you can protect your money is to review your bills.

5. Know when to ask for a second opinion. The Agency for Healthcare Research and Quality reports that 5% of all patents are misdiagnosed.[9] Getting the input of another physician can save you from unnecessary medical costs and procedure

6. Take advantage of free preventive care and health screenings. This is a no-cost way to stay on top of potential health issues.[10]

You should not be intimidated by medical professionals. They work for you.

Doctors and hospital are striving to deliver the right care at the right time in the right setting. However, they need you to help them. When you share your questions, concerns, and preferences, your care providers can be confident that you clearly understand your choices, and they can better help you coordinate any care and services.

Like anything else, the more you advocate for yourself the easier it will become. Finally, there is growing body of research that shows that passive patients are less likely to get well than people who take an active role in their care. You can help yourself to wellness by being active, communicating effectively, and engaging with your health care providers.

SECTION 2

Learn to Listen to Your Body

Tip: Pain and changes in your body's normal functions are two early warning signs you should not ignore.

If you are willing to pay attention to what your body is telling you, it's possible to find serious problems early. Many times, finding problems early results in less invasive and lower cost treatment, and a dramatic improvement in living a longer and healthier life.

Tip: Research shows that the survival rates of almost every major illness improve dramatically when the problem is found early, confined to its point of origin, and treated quickly.

Your body's warning signs can mean almost anything. They may be telling you to take a simple action like eat something, drink something, get some rest, change a habit, get some exercise, change your diet, stop reading books without glasses, or get new walking shoes.

Early warning signs may also mean that something is going wrong with your body's ability to perform its daily functions. When you feel warning signs that something may be wrong, pay attention. Consider if you have done anything that might be causing your body to react and whether any changes in your daily routine might be causing your symptoms.

If you think it is possible that your lifestyle might be causing your body to react, try to correct the problem yourself. For example, common heartburn can be caused by too much acid or sugar in your diet. Foot, ankle, knee, or hip pain might be caused by something as simple as wearing poor fitting shoes. Common headaches can be caused by stress, vision issues, allergies, diet issues, and simple dehydration.

Correcting a problem yourself can be as simple as making changes in your lifestyle. If you have tried solving the problem yourself without success, or if you feel that getting expert help is a better choice for you, then consider your options. Sometimes, finding health problems early is as simple as a basic screening test. Tests are often specialized for a specific disorder or a group of disorders. They are done for a variety of reasons.

The most common reasons for testing are to screen for illnesses before symptoms are present, to diagnose something that seems wrong, to evaluate the severity of a problem, and to monitor the response to a treatment. You can find more information about different tests in the *Merck Manual Consumer Version*, a widely used free publication. It can be accessed online at http://www.merckmanuals.com/home/appendixes/common-medical-tests/common-medical-tests.

Tests usually fall into one of the following categories:

Analysis of body fluids including blood, urine, spinal cord, brain, joints, sweat, saliva, and digestive fluids.

Imaging, which provides pictures inside your body. Examples are x-rays, MRI (magnetic resonance imaging) scans, PET (positron emission tomography) scans, CT (computerized tomography) scans, angiography, and radioisotope (nuclear) scans.

Endoscopy uses a camera on the end of a scope to view inside the body.

Body function measurement tests your heart's electrical activity or your lungs' ability to hold air.

Biopsy procedure that removes and examines small tissue samples for the presence of disease.

Genetic testing examines cells to check for abnormalities in chromosomes, including DNA.

Tip: One major advantage of screenings is to detect potential problems before you have symptoms, when lifestyle changes can be used to strengthen the body's natural ability to fight most problems.

The most common medical tests and screenings include the following:

Blood pressure: Normal blood pressure is less than 120/80 mm/Hg, according to the American Heart Association.[11] Blood pressure higher than 135/80 mm/Hg may result in the need for a hemoglobin A1C blood test or an oral glucose tolerance test. If your blood glucose is abnormally high, you may be diagnosed with diabetes.

Body mass index (BMI): The Centers for Disease Control and Prevention (CDC) say that an adult BMI between 18.5 and 25 is the normal range.[12]

Complete blood count (CBC): This blood test is used to diagnose numerous medical issues by measuring red blood cells, white blood cells, hemoglobin, and other aspects of your blood.

Prothrombin time (PT): This is a common blood test that measures how long it takes your blood to clot.

Cholesterol: The American Heart Association recommends that all adults 35 and older have their cholesterol checked every 5 years.[13] If you have any of the following risk factors, you should talk to your doctor about beginning screening earlier.

Risk factors include: diabetes, smoking, BMI over 30, family history of stoke, and close relatives who had a heart attack. The results will show your high-density lipoprotein, or HDL (good cholesterol) and low-density lipoprotein, or LDL (bad cholesterol). According to the Mayo Clinic, a healthy total cholesterol is below 200.[14]

Triglycerides: Often taken in conjunction with cholesterol testing, the triglyceride test can provide information about the amount of fat in your blood. Triglyceride levels below 150 mg/dL are considered normal. Optimal levels are less than 100 mg/dL.[15]

Colonoscopy: This test looks at your rectum and colon to detect early warning signs of cancer, unusual growths, and abnormalities. They are recommended for anyone older than 50 who has not been screened for colorectal cancer. You should consult your doctor about getting screened earlier if colorectal cancer runs in your family.[16] Colonoscopies are painless and take about 20 minutes.

Melanoma screening: These tests are conducted through visual examinations. They can and should be conducted by a self-skin exam and regular visits to a dermatologist. According to the American Cancer Society, more women get melanoma before age 50. However, by age 65, the ratio reverses. By age 80, men account for three times the number of new cases than women.[17]

Tip: Melanoma, like many other cancers today, is highly curable when detected early.

Pap smears: This test takes samples of cells from a women's cervix to look for changes that might indicate the presence of cervical cancer.

Mammography: This test uses x-rays to screen for tumors and breast cancer. It is usually recommended for women older than 40 and for younger women with increased risk factors.

Echocardiography: This painless test uses sound waves to make a moving picture of the heart chambers, valves, and surrounding structures. There is no exposure to radiation during this test.

Magnetic resonance imaging (MRI): MRIs use radio waves and magnetic fields to develop pictures of internal organs and structures like muscles, nerves, bones, and other tissue.

Computer axial tomography (CT or CAT scan): This scan is another type of x-ray that uses cross-sectional images to build detailed pictures of the inside of your body. Its primary uses are to let doctors find blood clots, tumors, infections, and other diseases and conditions.

Bone density study: This is a type of x-ray that is used to measure bone loss and diagnose osteoporosis.

Depression: There is no specific test for depression, an illness that affects many more people than we think. The National Institute of Mental Health estimates that 16 million people have at least one major depressive episode a year.[18]

Tip: If you're feeling down for more than a few weeks, consider speaking with your doctor. He or she will be able to help screen you and recommend treatments if needed.

It has become common for communities, hospitals, and health systems to hold free screening events and health fairs. Once you know what's available to you, speak with your doctor to determine what screening tests you need. Your doctor's recommendations will be based on your age, health, gender, risk factors, and lifestyle.

Risk factors are things that make getting a disease more likely. They may include your family's health history, your own lifestyle habits, and your symptoms. When you are considering getting a screening test, talk with your doctor about the following:

- What does the doctor hope to learn from the results?
- What are the costs of the test given your insurance?
- What is the test like?
- What are the risks and benefits of the test?
- How reliable is the test?
- What will the follow-up be?
- What are the alternatives to the test?
- What would happen if you chose not to have the test?

Tip: Screening tests are not 100% accurate in all cases, and every test has some risk.

Online Symptom Checkers

A second way that you can learn more about what your symptoms or body function changes are telling you is to try an online symptom checker.

It can't be stated strong enough or often enough that online symptom checkers, while useful to gather information, are never a substitute for a diagnosis from a qualified medical professional who has examined you in person.

A 2016 study by Harvard Medical School compared 23 different symptom checkers with pediatricians and internal medicine and family practice physicians for 45 different medical situations of varying complexity. Doctors made the correct diagnosis 72% of the time compared with 34% for online symptom checkers.[19]

The real value of an online symptom checker is to gather information that you can share with a doctor. However, as world-renowned e-patient Dave deBronkhart points out in his highly regarded blog, at http://www.epatientdave.com/blog/, do not bring in reams of paper and symptom checker information to your doctor. Your doctor will not have the time to review it all. A brief summary of what you found will do a much better job of helping your doctor diagnose the situation.

If you would like to try an online symptom checker, here is a brief list of leading resources:

AskMD
https://www.sharecare.com/askmd/get-started

Drugs.com
https://www.drugs.com/symptom-checker/

Everyday Health
https://www.everydayhealth.com/symptom-checker

Mayo Clinic
http://www.mayoclinic.org/symptom-checker/select-symptom/itt-20009075

WebMD
http://symptoms.webmd.com/#introView

A more traditional way to get answers about your symptoms is to schedule an appointment with your doctor, or another health professional, who is trained and experienced at successfully treating your symptoms.

Tip: Nurses and doctors often have a lot of knowledge about other doctors and health care professionals who do excellent work. If you have a serious diagnosis, don't hesitate to ask them who they would trust to help them if they were in your shoes. They may or may not provide an answer. However, you have very little to lose by asking.

When you need to find a doctor or specialist, obtain a list of qualified physicians in your area. Your insurance company is a great starting point. If you are uninsured, your state health department is another option. From that list, choose a few physician offices to contact. Additional guidelines for finding lists and choosing physicians are discussed in Section 6 of this *Guide*.

When you first speak to someone from the physician's office, introduce yourself and explain your situation. Then ask the following:

- Does the practice accept your insurance?
- How much experience does the physician have treating people with symptoms like yours?
- If the person scheduling your appointment knows what will be done during the first appointment?
- If any tests or procedures will be done during your appointment?
- What you need to bring to the appointment?
- What forms need to be completed prior to your appointment, how much time it usually takes to complete the forms, and if there is a website where you can print and complete them before you come in for your appointment?
- How much time the doctor or health provider will have to spend with you?
- How much will you have to pay out of pocket for the appointment and any tests that the doctor might want to perform?
- If the doctor will be available to answer any questions you might have after the appointment and how long it usually takes to get answers?

If you feel that the people at the practice are not responsive to your questions, or if they seem annoyed by your questions, ask if there is a better time to discuss your situation. If they say yes, find a better time and call back.

If the initial call isn't going well, remember that it just may be that the person representing the practice is having a bad moment at the time of your call. It may also mean that the practice is not patient friendly. If the latter is the case, you should consider calling the next practice on your list. Although your first experience may not reflect the nature of the practice, you will get the best care from a provider who will listen to you and understand your concerns and preferences.

Your Initial Doctor Appointment

Visiting a doctor's office can make anyone nervous and even scared. You may have only a few minutes with the doctor to discuss your concerns. To make sure that you have the information you need by the end of your first appointment, follow the steps below:

Step 1: Explain Your Condition

Prepare a list of questions for the doctor before the appointment. See Sections 6 and 8 in this *Guide* for suggested questions. Consider writing down your symptoms, any recent changes in your condition, and anything that seems out of the ordinary.

Questions to ask yourself about your symptoms include:

- What exactly are my symptoms?
- Are the symptoms constant, or how often do I experience them?

- Does anything I do make the symptoms better or worse?
- Do the symptoms affect my daily activities, and if so, which ones and how?

Step 2: Ask Doctor for Forms

If possible, ask the doctor's office to send you any forms that need to be filled out and complete them before arriving for the appointment. You may also be able to do this on the practice's website. Make a list of your prescription and over-the-counter drugs, supplements, and vitamins. If you don't make a list, bring the medicines and supplements with you to your appointment.

Step 3: Make a List of Your Concerns

Take your list of concerns with you when you meet with your doctor.

Tip: Contact your insurance provider and/or Medicare/Medicaid and find out:

- *What your insurance will pay for, and how much you'll have to pay.*
- *If your doctor is in your network or not. For your first appointment, find a doctor who is covered in your insurance plan network. Additional steps for finding the right doctor for you are detailed in Section 6.*

What You Should Do for an Initial Appointment

- Get the most recent copy of your insurance plan.
- Ask the doctor's office to send you a copy of any forms that the practice wants completed before your visit. If they're available on the practice website, fill them out before your appointment. If you have problems understanding how to fill out any of the forms, call the practice and ask for help. Some community organizations also provide this kind of help.
- Do whatever you need to ensure that you can focus on the doctor. It's critical to understand and remember important information. If your memory isn't that great, you might use a small tape recorder during the visit or bring a family member or friend to take notes. Bring an interpreter if you know you'll need one.

Tip: If you need a tape recorder or other help, let the doctor know beforehand.

Most doctors will not have any problem with you recording an appointment or bringing another person. However, some will get defensive. If happens doctor becomes defensive, don't let it stop you from working with him or her. Just make sure that you write down as much as you can about any tests, diagnosis, or treatment plans.

Your first meeting is a good time to talk with the doctor and the office staff about some communication basics. When you see the doctor and office staff, introduce yourself and let them know by what name you like to be called. For example: "Hello, my name is Mrs. Smith," or

"Good morning, my name is Bob Jones. Please call me Bob."

Ask how the office runs. Learn what days are busiest and what times are best to call. Ask what to do if there is an emergency, or if you need a doctor when the office is closed. If you haven't already, you may have to fill out some forms, including your medical history, insurance information, personal information, and a medical release form.

Talking about your health means sharing information about how you feel physically, emotionally, and mentally. Knowing how to describe your symptoms and bringing up other concerns will help you become a partner with your health care providers.

Discuss any symptoms you are having. A symptom is evidence of something that may be going wrong in your body. Examples of symptoms include dizziness, trouble breathing, pain, fever, a lump or bump, unexplained weight loss or gain, having a hard time sleeping, or anything that seems different from your normal body functions. Be clear and concise when describing your symptoms. Your description helps the doctor identify the problem. A physical exam and medical tests will provide valuable information too, but it is your symptoms that point the doctor in the right direction.

Your doctor should ask when your symptoms started, what time of day they happen, how long they last, how often they occur, if they seem to be getting worse or better, and if they keep you from going out or doing your usual activities. Worrying about your symptoms is not a sign of weakness. Being honest about what you are experiencing doesn't mean that you are complaining. The doctor needs to know how you feel.

Give the doctor information about your medications, supplements, and vitamins. It is possible for medicines to interact and cause unpleasant and sometimes dangerous side effects. The easiest way to give your doctor this information is to write down your medications, how often you take them, and what doses you take. You can even take pictures of the labels with a smartphone, digital camera, or mobile device.

Your doctor needs to know about ALL the medicines you take, including over-the-counter (nonprescription) drugs and herbal remedies or supplements. It can't hurt to bring your medications with you to your first appointment, and don't forget about eye drops, vitamins, and laxatives. Describe any reactions you have had. Tell your doctor which medications work best for you.

Tip: If you use a specific pharmacy, tell the doctor.

Also, tell the doctor about your habits. To provide the best care possible, your doctor should understand you as a person and know what your life is like. The doctor may ask questions about where you live, what you eat, how you sleep, what you do each day, what activities you enjoy, what your sex life is like, and if you smoke or drink. Be open and honest with your doctor. It will help him or her understand your medical condition(s) fully and recommend the best treatment choices for you.

Voice any concerns you have. Your doctor may ask you a general question like "how is your life going?" This is not being impolite or nosy. Information about what is happening in your life may be useful medically.

Let the doctor know about any major changes or stress in your life, such as a divorce or the death of a loved one. You don't have to go into detail. You may want to say something like, "It might be helpful for you to know that my father died since the last time we talked," or "I recently bought a new house and my mother moved in with me."

Tip: Don't forget to research and bring your previous doctors' names and contact information. This will help your new doctor get copies of your medical records.

Before Leaving the Initial Appointment

Find out how to get your questions answered after you have left the doctor's office, as well as after-hours when the office is closed.

Tip: If you didn't request copies of your records, tests, and doctor's notes when you checked in, do that before you leave.

Federal laws require doctors, hospitals, and medical providers to provide you with copies of your medical records, although you may have to pay a small fee. Ask how much you will be expected to pay, and what the procedures are for getting your copies.

Tip: You need to be 100% clear about any next steps suggested by your doctor before you leave.

Tip: Be polite with the office staff, even if they are not so nice to you. You may need their help some day.

Heeding Early Warning Signs

Early warning signs are almost always trying to tell you something. The challenges are learning to listen to what your body is trying to tell you, understanding what those warning signs or symptoms mean, and taking the appropriate action.

The most common reasons that life-threatening illnesses are not diagnosed early are that people do not know the early warning signs or symptoms, or they ignore them. Other reasons for delayed diagnosis include not scheduling a doctor's appointment out of fear of finding out what's wrong, concerns over the costs of treatment, and delays in getting tests.

Do not make your situation worse by ignoring early warning signs and symptoms, or letting fear or cost stop you from seeking help. If you choose to do nothing about your symptoms, make sure that it's because you have consulted with your doctor, you fully understand the consequences, and you have decided that doing nothing is in your best interest.

SECTION 3

You're Sick or Hurt . . . What Now?

The Early Steps

You just got the news from your doctor that you're sick, and it's a life-threatening or chronic illness. What now?

As soon as you balance your emotions, you'll have to make important decisions about your diagnosis, doctors, treatment, care, and finances. During the next few days, weeks, and months, you must learn enough about your choices to make informed decisions. It's your right and responsibility if you want safe, quality health care.

While you need never walk the path to wellness alone, you must walk it. If you choose not to work with your health care team and accept responsibility for yourself, you will be at the mercy of a broken health care system. The path to safe, quality, and affordable health care is paved with obstacles that you need to get around, over, and through. Trust in your health care providers, verify everything, and consider your preferences above all.

Maybe, your doctor or insurance provider has already provided you information in the form of a pamphlet, website, or video specific to your diagnosis. However, it's likely to take a little time before you process your new diagnosis and are ready to make good decisions. There are a wide range of emotions that people might feel after getting a serious diagnosis. Those emotions include anger, helplessness, depression, confusion, and fear to name a few.

It's important that you realize that these feelings are natural. Grief can also be a major factor for anyone after being diagnosed with a serious or life-threatening illness.

The Swiss American psychologist Elisabeth Kubler-Ross developed a model known as the Five Stages of Grief. They are:

1. Denial: "This can't be happening."
2. Anger: "Why me? This is not fair!"
3. Bargaining: "Please let me live until my children are grown."
4. Depression: "Why bother with anything—I'm going to die anyway."
5. Acceptance: "It's going to be alright."[20]

Grieving is not necessarily a linear process, and you may not experience each stage in the manner outlined by Kubler-Ross. What matters is that there are steps you can take to control your feelings, balance yourself, and self-advocate for the safest and best health care possible.

Step 1. Understand Your Emotions

It is common to feel shock, anger, frustration, worry, and other emotions when you are told you that you have a life-threatening or serious illness. It's even common to experience short-term changes in your behavior after hearing such serious news. Usually, your emotions and any behavioral changes are temporary. They typically start returning to normal within weeks when you have support.

You can help yourself balance your emotions as soon as possible by finding someone you trust to talk to. If there is no one in your life who you trust that much, consider seeking out and communicating with others who have experienced a similar diagnosis. Often, other patients are able to fully understand what you're going through. Sometimes the comfort of being anonymous also lets you express your feelings to others who you hardly know because you have shared a common experience.

Support groups are also available in many online communities. A list of online patient communities is included later in this section, in Section 10 of this *Guide*, and online at www.aPatientsPlace.com.

Tip: Make every effort to visit and participate in a patient chat room or online Q&A.

Tip: Trust, but verify everything you learn in chat rooms with your physicians.

Tip: While great new physician-patient communication solutions are on the way, it's the responsibility of each patient or their caregiver to ensure that doctors and health providers have access to all past appointment notes and other clinically relevant information.

You'll make better choices after your emotions settle down. It is not advisable to make any immediate decisions regarding your health after a serious diagnosis unless your doctor tells you that you must act quickly. If you must make a quick decision, try to get a second opinion beforehand. If your reactions to the news do not get better within a few weeks or if they get worse, ask your doctor about mental health counselors and support that is available.

Step 2. Take Control

Why do some people seem to continue on with their lives, and others seem to make their lives all about their illness? Why do some people recover quickly and others not? Why do some people seem to resume active and productive lives and others not? Although the answers are not simple, we have learned that you can influence your outcomes through your actions.

Make no mistake, your choices about your health care and your lifestyle are scientifically proven to affect how likely you are to minimize the effects of your illness and maximize your chances of achieving the best recovery possible. Your choices may mean the difference between returning to health or not. You are not a victim. You are normal, like everybody else.

The majority of people in the world are going to be diagnosed with a major illness or disease during their life. When it's happens to you, remember that there are a lot of people who have been in your shoes and others who are currently walking a similar path in their lives. You are not alone.

Step 3. Schedule a Follow-Up Appointment

As soon as you can after your diagnosis, schedule a follow-up appointment with your doctor or specialist. If you are going to see a specialist, let your primary physician know. During the follow-up appointment you will want to discuss the diagnosis, ask questions, and learn your options.

Tip: When you call to schedule a follow up appointment after your diagnosis, tell your doctor's scheduling person that you would like a little extra time with the doctor to ensure that you understand your circumstances and choices.

While you are waiting for your follow-up appointment, do the following:

- Take time to talk to friends, family, and other patients about your feelings.
- Learn the basics about your illness; see Step 6 below.
- Contact your insurance provider to inform them of the diagnosis, ask if the expenses of a second opinion are covered, ask what expenses you will be expected to pay yourself, and request a case manager.
- Prepare your list of questions for the doctor; see Step 9 below.

Step 4. Find Support

As mentioned earlier, it's very important that you find someone you trust to talk to about your feelings and choices. If you can find a few people, that's even better. If you don't have anyone in your life whom you trust enough to discuss intimate issues, you can seek support online from the patient groups listed below, from the local chapter of the professional organization for your illness, or from the list of patient communities at www.aPatientsPlace.com. Even if you don't contact the people in these communities right away, sign on and read what they are saying to one another.

Online Patient Communities

www.aPatientsPlace.com
Click on the "Connect to Other Patients" icon near the top of the home page to go to a large index of patient-to-patient chat rooms.

www.patientslikeme.com
This site allows patients to record data about themselves and share it in an open environment. Patients can identify others with similar illnesses at similar stages. They can also share their experiences with treatments and medications.

www.MDJunction.com
This site offers patient communities with almost exclusively patient-driven content.

www.acor.org
The Association of Cancer Online Resources has over 140 communities to share information and support.

www.dailystrength.org
This site has support groups in a multitude of categories; it is not exclusively for illnesses.

Step 5. Keep as Many of Your Daily Routines as Possible

A serious diagnosis can bring a great deal of uncertainty into your life, and possibly into the lives of your family and close friends as well. The familiarity of continuing as many of your usual routines and activities as possible helps everyone, including yourself, feel more secure.

Step 6. Learn about Your Illness

You will maximize your time and your doctor(s)' if you educate yourself about your illness before you have a follow-up appointment.

Tip: You shouldn't expect your doctor or any other medical professional to know everything about your illness. According to Dr. Donald Lindberg, the former director of the National Library of Medicine, "If I read two new journal articles every night, at the end of a year I'd be 400 years behind."[21]

If you have Internet access at home, go to a reliable source of information. Reliable sources for starting your search are listed below. Do not expect to find everything about your illness by yourself. If you can learn about the nature of the illness and its usual treatment, you will be well prepared to ask your doctor about the things that are on your mind and to listen to the answers.

Start your search on a trustworthy website from an organization that also reviews the quality of the websites and information it links to. Some of the very best are:

www.healthfinder.gov
Healthfinder, from the U.S. Department of Health and
Human Services, offers health information that has been
reviewed by professionals, as well as websites, medical
groups, a medical dictionary, drug information, and much
more.

http://www.nlm.nih.gov/medlineplus
MedlinePlus is from the National Institutes of Health. You
can search more than 800 health topics, prescription and
over-the-counter drugs, news, professional directories, local
resources, and a medical encyclopedia with images. Health
information is available in dozens of languages.

Other trusted and reliable health websites are:

www.WebMD.com
WebMD is a highly trafficked health portal.

www.MedicineNet.com
MedicineNet is owned and operated by WebMD. The site
provides in-depth medical information produced by a
network of more than 70 U.S. board certified physicians.

If you want detailed information from the latest articles
and medical research in medical journals, visit these
websites:

https://www.ncbi.nlm.nih.gov/pubmed/ PubMed is the
National Library of Medicine's database of references to
more than 14 million articles published in 4,800 medical
and scientific journals. Read the summaries (abstracts) first
to determine if you should get a copy of or read the entire
article. The article might be free, or it might require a fee
charged by the publisher.

www.pubmedcentral.nih.gov
PubMed Central is the National Library of Medicine's database of journal articles that are available free of charge to users.

An expanded list of health websites is included in Addendum 4 of this *Guide* and online at www.aPatientsPlace.com.

Researching your illness through the resources listed above should provide you with a basic understanding of:

- The nature of your illness.
- How the illness normally affects people.
- The specialist(s) who typically treat the illness.
- What the standard treatments are.
- What the common prognosis (expected outcome) is.

As soon as you understand these basics about your illness, you will be able to prepare questions for your doctor, and you will also be able to evaluate whether the answers help you understand your choices.

Step 7. Learn about Your Insurance

Tip: Call your insurance provider and get a copy of your insurance plan.

When you purchased health insurance or applied for public aide, you agreed to abide by the rules of the plan or program. To avoid misunderstandings about your coverage, you need to do the following:

- Read your insurance plan or program guidelines.

- Contact your insurance company or program manager and discuss your situation with a service representative before you go back to your doctor or a specialist.

When you call an insurance or program customer service phone number, do the following:

- Get the name of the person you are speaking to.
- Make sure you have an up-to-date copy of your plan or program guidelines.
- Keep a record of the day and time you speak with the representatives and what was said.
- Explain your recent diagnosis.
- Ask how to file a claim.
- Ask for a case manager to be assigned to your case so that you may speak with the same person all the time throughout the diagnosis, treatment, and care of your condition.

Tip: If the person who you are speaking with refuses to give you the name of a case manager, ask to speak with a manager.

- Ask what expenses will be covered under your plan and what might not be covered.
- Ask what expenses you should expect to pay yourself. Don't forget to ask if a second opinion, additional diagnostic testing, and all treatments are covered under your personal policy.

For additional step-by-step instructions about how to work with your insurance providers, go to Section 4 in this *Guide,* "Working with Your Insurance Provider."

Step 8. Prepare for Your Follow-up Appointment

If you don't ask questions, you won't have the information you need to make good choices, and your doctor may feel that she or he has answered all your questions in a manner that you understand. Your doctor may also feel that you don't want any more information.

Tip: Prepare your questions in advance, and plan to write down or record the answers so you don't forget anything.

The suggested questions below are a guideline to help you. You may have others of your own. The answers should give you a better understanding of your situation and choices. The most important goal is to have all of the information you need to consider clearly what is in your best interest.

Suggested questions for primary care doctors and specialists should cover the following areas:

- Your illness or condition.
- The tests used to diagnose your illness or condition, and traditional, new, and nonstandard treatments for your illness or condition.
- Your insurance coverage and financial obligations.
- Recommended resources for additional information support.

Questions to Ask a Primary Care Physician

Q. What tests were used to diagnose my condition, and what did they show you?

You should learn the technical name of the tests that your doctor used or plans to use to make a diagnosis, get copies of the results, and find out what led the doctor to his or her diagnosis.

Q. What is the technical name of my disease or illness?

You should learn the technical name and the practical nature of your illness.

Q. How does the disease or illness affect my body, and how should I expect this to change over time?

You should learn what people experience in most cases, both in the near and long-term future.

Q. What is my prognosis (outlook for the future) with and without treatment?

You should learn what to expect in terms of your ability to function, quality of life, and expected interactions with health care providers during your treatment, and what you could expect if you did not pursue any treatment at all.

Q. Can you refer me to any specialists?

You should learn if your doctor knows any specialists for your condition, specifically someone the doctor has worked with before.

Questions to Ask a Specialist

Q. Will I need any additional tests? If the answer is no, move on to the next questions. If the answer is yes, ask these follow-up questions:

- What are the names of the tests?
- What will each test show?
- What are the risks of each test?
- What should I expect on before, during, and after the tests?
- Will I feel any pain?
- Will I need to be medicated or sedated for each test?
- Are there any alternatives to the tests?
- Are the tests routinely covered by my insurance?
- How can I learn more about each test?

Based on the answers to the questions above, you should learn what additional test(s) you might need to take, the basic nature of each test, what the specialist hopes to find out from each test, and the specialist's perspective of how each treatment option will affect you.

Other questions that you might ask include:

Q. What are the standard and new treatment options for my condition?

Q. What are the pros and cons of each treatment option?

Q. Which treatment do you recommend for me? Why?

Q. Will my insurance cover the costs of the treatments?

Q. Are you aware of or do you recommend any alternative or complimentary treatments?

You should learn if the specialist has any familiarity with alternative and complimentary medicine. If the specialist is comfortable discussing this with you, you may find other treatment options to look into.

Q. How soon do I need to make a decision about treatment?

You should learn how much time the specialist feels you have to consider your treatment alternatives. If he or she wants you to immediately have a major surgical procedure or treatment that is invasive and/or irreversible, you must find out why, what will happen if you don't have the procedure or treatment immediately, and how quickly you can get a second opinion from another specialist?

Q. Are there clinical trials that may be right for me?

You should learn if the specialist is familiar with any clinical trials, both locally and nationally, that you would qualify for, and if he or she would recommend your participation.

Q. Now that I have this diagnosis, what changes will I need to make in my daily life?

You should learn if and how your illness will affect your activities and routines, any additional tests that may be needed, and how any treatments will impact your living situation, your quality of life, and your finances.

Q. Do you know if insurance usually covers the treatment you are recommending?

You should learn if the recommended treatment is usually covered by insurance.

Q. Will you help me try to get my insurance to pay for whatever treatment and rehabilitation I decide is right for me?

You should learn if the specialist will help you obtain coverage from your insurance company if you choose a new, experimental, or alternative treatment.

Q. How can I get copies of my medical records?

You should learn the procedures are for getting copies of your records and test results.

Since most people typically remember less than 10% of what they hear, you may want to consider what would be the most comfortable and effective way to ensure that you remember the answers you're given. One option is simply to write the answers down on a piece of paper. If you feel you may be so busy writing that you are going to miss something, consider bringing a small cassette recorder or another person with you. Just make sure you tell your doctor(s) what you're doing beforehand so they are not surprised.

Whatever you do, make sure you that you are informed of and understand your options. This is your legal right and obligation. If you are unclear about anything, make sure that you have a way to follow up until you are clear about your choices.

Step 9. Get Copies of Your Medical Records and Test Results

It's much easier to get copies of your medical records if you request them when you first visit your doctor's office or treatment facility versus trying to get them after you have left. When you call to schedule your appointment, ask about the policies and costs for obtaining copies of your medical records and test results. Most providers will have you fill out a standard form when you get to their office for your scheduled appointment.

If your appointment is not scheduled for a week or more, or you find out that your doctor's office does not have a standard form, submit your written request for copies to your doctor as soon as you can. You should expect to be charged reasonable fees for the office's time and the copies. If for any reason you can't afford to pay the fees, discuss your situation with your doctor immediately. Most doctors will not allow you to take your records and copy them yourself.

Keep in mind that if you want copies of any imaging tests, such as x-rays or MRIs, it may cost more. Ask the office when you could reasonably expect the copies to be ready for pickup, and set a date to get them. On the date that your records are ready, bring with you to the doctor's office a copy of your medical release and a check for the full amount of the copies.

If you need to write a letter requesting your records, you can use the sample letter in Addendum 1 of this *Guide* as a draft. At the beginning of your request letter you will need to specify:

- The medical provider's name
- The medical provider's address
- Your name
- Your address
- Your medical record or case number (you can get this from the office staff).
- Social Security number and insurance ID number).
- The specific dates that you received service.

Be specific about what records you want. Do you want billing information included? Do you want the provider's handwritten notes or typed reports, or your test results? Under most circumstances, providers have 30 days from the date they receive your written request to get you copies. Since you will often want them quicker than that, be kind, considerate, and persistent with your doctor's office staff.

Step 10. Consult an Experienced Specialist

When you are diagnosed or suspect that you may be diagnosed with a serious illness, injury, or condition, one of the most important things that you should do is to consult a board certified specialist with experience treating your condition. Just make sure to speak with your health insurance provider first so you understand what is covered by your policy, what financial obligations you will have, and what rules or processes that you need to follow to ensure maximum financial coverage.

Tip: Once your original diagnosis is confirmed by a second specialist, the likelihood that the diagnosis is accurate is much higher.

Step 11. The Second Follow-up Appointment

During the follow-up appointment, you should expect your doctor to help you understand your diagnosis, discuss whether more tests are recommended, discus your treatment options, answer your questions, and develop a treatment plan that you agree with. You should also be able to decide if you feel your doctor will be a good partner in fighting your illness or condition.

Make sure that by the time you leave, you have a good understanding of your diagnosis and potential treatment options. Ask for any instructions given to you to be written down. If you still have trouble understanding them, ask where you can go for more information.

When you leave the doctor, you need to be prepared to investigate and ultimately make decisions about your doctor and treatment. Before you begin any treatment you should consider whether you want another opinion (this is discussed in the next step), whether the doctor you have met with is the right one for you to work with, and what treatment is right for you.

Step 12. Confirm Your Diagnosis

The first diagnosis is not always the correct diagnosis. Remember that a diagnosis is what your doctor thinks is wrong. Although, doctors are well trained and often very experienced, there are millions of misdiagnosed patients and tens of thousands of preventable deaths in the United States each year.[22]

In order to confirm your diagnosis, you should get copies of your medical records and possibly a second opinion. If you get a second opinion that is different from the original diagnosis, you should call your insurance provider and request coverage for a third opinion from an expert in your illness or condition.

Step 13. Get a Second and Even a Third Opinion

You should get a second opinion in all cases when you are diagnosed with a major illness or condition. This is important because you have to be confident that you know beyond a doubt what illness or condition you are dealing with and what your options are in order to make good treatment decisions. Many times your insurance provider will require a second opinion before approving payment for a costly treatment.

Since doctors are viewed by most people as trusting, caring, and honest, it's easy for patients to feel that their doctor will be offended if they tell him or her that they would like the opinion of another doctor. Do not let this feeling prevent you from getting a second opinion. Doctors should be comfortable with their patients seeking the opinion of another doctor. In most cases, they should encourage it.

A second opinion is probably a good idea if you are:

- Diagnosed with a life-threatening illness or condition.
- Told you need a major surgery or an invasive test.
- Not completely confident in the original diagnosis.

- Feeling that you need to speak with a doctor who is an expert at treating your illness or condition.
- Unhappy that your regular doctor can't diagnose your problem.
- Having trouble talking with your current doctors.
- Not seeing improvement in your medical condition.
- Told a second surgery is recommended.
- Having multiple medical problems.

If possible, try to meet face-to-face with the doctor providing the second opinion. There are great hospitals such as the Mayo Clinic that will give you their expert opinion based on reviewing your tests and records, too. While this can be valuable, it is not the same as seeing the doctor in person. Make sure you write down all of your questions for the doctor providing the second opinion. You may also want to have someone you trust, maybe even your first doctor, review your questions. You will also need copies of your medical records sent to the second doctor.

If a diagnosis from a second specialist is different than the diagnosis from the first specialist, take the steps below to help you sort out what is going on.

Step 1. Find a Specialist

Tell your primary care doctor that you would like the name of another specialist so you can get a third opinion, to clarify the differences in the initial diagnosis and second opinion. Any doctor worthy of the practice of medicine will be supportive. If your doctor is not supportive, that is a warning sign that you most definitely need a third opinion.

Tip: Be careful that your doctor does not simply refer a friend or colleague. You want your doctor to recommend someone who is an expert at treating your condition, not just someone your doctor has a personal friendship with.

You should not look for a specialist that your primary care doctor plays golf with. If you need to find an expert on your own, go to Section 6 in this *Guide* titled "Finding the Right Doctors and Health Providers" and follow the instructions.

Do not go to another doctor from the same practice as the initial doctor for a second opinion unless you are 100% confident that the doctor you are being referred to is a bona fide expert. Check with your health insurance provider to find out if t you have coverage for a second or third opinion. Find out what procedures you or your first doctor need to follow to ensure that your provider pays for the second and third opinion.

Step 2: Handle Your Medical Records

Ask to have your medical records sent from your initial doctor to your new doctor. Follow the steps provided earlier in this section to have those copies sent to your new doctor, and be sure to get copies for your own records.

Step 3 Get Your Questions Together

Write down the questions you want answered, and make sure you get very specific answers. One of the most important questions you need to ask is whether your doctor has all of the information he or she needs to issue a second opinion. The questions you want to ask the doctor providing the second opinion are different than the questions you asked your first doctor. Use the list of questions below as a guide:

Q. What is the likelihood that my medical problem could have a different diagnosis than the one I was given?

Q. What are the traditional and alternative forms of treatment for my condition?

Q. Which treatment typically has the best results?

Q. What are the likely outcomes if I wait or if I don't have the recommended treatment?

Q. What are the risks associated with each possible treatment?

Q. Are there any side effects or residual effects from each treatment option?

Q. How will each treatment improve my health or the quality of my life?

Q. How long is the recovery period?

If the second opinion differs from the initial one, or if the second doctor is not confident with your original diagnosis, you will want to know why. It's important to understand the reasoning behind a medical opinion. You should leave that appointment knowing if additional tests might help to provide a clearer understanding of your condition, and your treatment options. This information will be critical should you seek a third opinion. Most important, make sure that you get a written copy of the second doctor's findings, and that you know who to call if you have any questions after reviewing that report.

Step 4. Learn as Much as You Can about Your illness or Condition

Review sections 6, 10, 11, and 12 in Volumes 2 and 3 of this *Guide* for step-by-step instructions on how to research your condition, learn about treatment options, find qualified doctors and hospitals, access clinical trials, connect with patient groups, and find local resources and support.

Remote Second Opinions

In today's medical system, you can also get a remote second opinion from experts at leading medical institutions. Insurance often won't pay for online second opinions, so make sure you understand the costs up front. Some of the providers include:

MyConsult Online Medical Second Opinion
(https://my.clevelandclinic.org/online-services/myconsult). This group is affiliated with the world-renowned Cleveland Clinic. At the time of writing this *Guide*, the group charged $565 for an online second opinion. If a pathologist was needed (with cancer this is usually the case), there was an additional charge of $180.

Partners Online Second Opinion
(https://econsults.partners.org). This group is affiliated with Partners HealthCare, a Harvard Medical School—affiliated health care delivery system. The group draws on the collective expertise of the physicians at all of the Partners'

hospitals, which include Brigham and Women's Hospital, Massachusetts General Hospital, and Dana-Farber/Partners Cancer Care. At the time of writing this *Guide* the basic cost for a specialist's opinion was $495. If needed, radiology and pathology reviews were an additional $200 and $250, respectively.

As you take each step on your journey to well-being, remember that research shows that patients who are more involved in their health care tend to get better results and be more satisfied.

SECTION 4

Working with Insurance Providers

Need Free Help Fast?

For no cost, you can contact the Patient Advocate Foundation (PAF) to help you solve your insurance issues. The PAF employs case managers to help people with financial, insurance, access, and employment-related issues relating to chronic, debilitating, and life-threatening illnesses. You can contact the PAF by calling 1-800-532-5274, by email at help@patientadvocate.org, and by visiting their website at www.patientadvocate.org.

For issues related to Medicare or Medicaid, you can call the Medicare Rights Center phone hotline from 9:00 a.m. to 5:00 p.m. Eastern time at 1-800-333-4114, or the official Medicare information line 24 hours a day, 7 days a week at 1-800-633-4227.

Health Insurance Basics

Today, health insurance helps pay for some of the medical costs associated with prevention, certain health screenings, basic illnesses, and many major conditions. However, it is highly likely that you will still have out-of-pocket costs. When you add your out-of-pocket expenses to your monthly premium, which is the amount you pay every month for your policy, you can figure out about how much you will have to spend on your health care.

Before you start comparing policies, it helps to know a few key terms:

Premium: The monthly amount you pay for your policy.

Deductible: How much money you will have to pay each year before the policy coverage starts.

Co-pay: The amount you have to pay for services.

Co-insurance: The percentage of the total charges that you have to pay in addition to your co-pay.

Out-of-pocket maximum: The top amount you can spend outside the premium during the benefit year.

Today, consumers are paying more of their medical expenses through higher premiums, higher deductibles, and higher co-insurance. To control your costs, it's important to know exactly what your health insurance plan covers and what it does not. For most insurance plans, the important rules fall into the following groups:

Doctors and Hospitals

Insurance companies sign contracts with doctors, hospitals, and other health care professionals to care for their plan members. Your plan likely refers to these groups as providers. In return the contracted doctors, hospitals, and other providers agree to certain reimbursement rates for the services they provide, and they agree to follow the plan's rules. This group of providers is often called the plan's network.

Tip: Your insurance company might not pay for you to go to a provider who is not in its network, or it may pay much less. You are responsible for the part of the bill that the plan doesn't pay.

Even if your doctor is part of the plan's network, he or she may prefer to send patients to a hospital that is not in the network. If that happens, ask if your doctor can send you to a hospital in your network. If that's not possible, you can ask the insurance company if it will approve the use of the out-of-network hospital. If no other arrangements can be made, you might have to choose a different doctor who has privileges at a hospital that is in your network. Your insurance company customer service can help you find qualified doctors who practice at in-network hospitals and treatment facilities.

Rules for Seeing Specialists

Many managed care plans, especially health maintenance organizations (HMOs), will not pay for you to see a specialist unless your primary care physician thinks it is necessary. If you see a specialist without a referral from your physician, you might have to pay for it out-of-pocket. These rules may be different if your plan is a preferred provider organization (PPO), where physician referrals are not required. .

Rules for Getting Expensive Services

If your doctor decides that you need to go to the hospital, have surgery, or have certain tests, your insurance company may refuse to pay for it unless it can preauthorize the treatment (approve it beforehand).

Medicines

Almost every managed care plan has a drug formulary. A formulary is a list of prescription medicines that your health plan has approved. If a drug isn't on the formulary, you will probably have to pay more for it. Your insurance company can give you a list of drugs that are on its formulary. If necessary, show the list to your doctor when he or she writes you a prescription.

Choosing a Health Insurance Plan

Step 1. Understand the Details of Each Policy

If you don't understand the details of a policy, call the health insurance company and ask for an explanation of how much money you will be responsible for paying on each plan you are considering. Make sure to ask about your monthly payment, deductible, and co-insurance, and get a list of benefits (what is covered and what is not).

Step 2. Calculate Your Expected Annual Cost for Each Policy

Calculate your health costs for the coming year to see whether you are better off with a high deductible and lower monthly premium or a low deductible and higher monthly premium. The way to do this is to add the amount of money you spent out-of-pocket on prescriptions, doctors' appointments, and medical devices and equipment in the past year or two and compare that with the co-payments and/or co-insurance offered by the plans you are considering.

If you choose a high-deductible option, consider using a health savings account (HSA) to set aside pretax dollars to pay for medical expenses. HSAs are explained later in this section. You must record your use of this account and keep detailed records. Add the expenses for all of the people who will be covered by the policy. As best you can, consider any additional or likely expenses for the upcoming year.

Step 3. Compare Costs of Each Policy

Based on the type of services you expect to need, compare the costs of using doctors and hospitals that are in the plan's network versus those not in the network. Check the maximum out-of-pocket amount to see whether the

deductible, co-payments, and prescription costs can be
applied toward it.

Step 4. Compare the Performance of Each Policy

Many health care organizations, such as the nonprofit
National Committee for Quality Assurance (NCQA), gather
data on how well doctors and facilities in health care plans
follow practice guidelines. It uses the results to grade,
accredit, and recognize those practices and facilities. To see
how your health plan and others in your area fare, go to
www.ncqa.org.

Another resource to help you select a health plan is the
Agency for Healthcare Research and Quality (AHRQ)
CAHPS database of health plan surveys. Using this
resource, you can review consumer surveys of health plans,
including Medicare and Medicaid. The survey information
can be accessed by the public at
https://cahpsdatabase.ahrq.gov/CAHPSIDB/default.aspx.
Experts hope that eventually the grades will extend all the
way down to practice groups and even individual
physicians.

Working with Your Insurance Company

Health insurance plans can be confusing. However, you
are responsible for knowing what benefits you are entitled
to under your policy. If you do not fully understand

something, ask your insurance representative or your employer's benefits administrator to explain it.

Following the steps below will help ensure that you receive all the benefits to which you're entitled.

- Make sure you have accurate contact information for your insurance company.
- Contact your insurance provider and request an up-to-date copy of your plan and its summary.

This will tell you how your plan works, covered benefits, and how to file a claim. Be confident when calling your insurance company. You are their customer. You have the right to receive complete information regarding your health benefits.

Your insurance company's customer service representatives are there to assist you. Part of their job includes answering questions to your satisfaction. Communicate as clearly and calmly as possible. Be courteous and polite, even if you are not happy with your insurance provider. The person on the other end of the phone probably wasn't responsible for whatever has disappointed you. Remember that your ultimate goal is to get coverage for what you need.

If you are met with resistance, simply restate your request. Carefully follow the steps outlined by your health plan for requesting prior authorization, submitting claims, or filing appeals. Not following these steps may result in a delay in processing or a denial of your request for coverage.

Tip: Don't give up. Don't take no for an answer.

If you have tried discussing your request with your health plan's customer service representative but are not satisfied with how your insurance matter was handled, ask to speak to a supervisor in the customer service department, or the manager or director of customer service or member services.

Follow up in writing or email after speaking with a health plan representative on the phone. Keep your correspondence simple and to the point. Include relevant dates, names of representatives with whom you spoke, and what was discussed. Also be sure to include your name, policy number, and any other identifying information. Do not hesitate to ask for help from your employer's human resources department or your health care provider.

In many cases, your employer makes decisions about what will be covered under your health plan. Your employer's support can also influence the approval of your request for coverage. Having your doctor contact your insurance representative can also be helpful since she or her can support the communication that you have had with your insurance company as to why the requested medical products or services are needed.

Advocate for yourself at all times. If needed, write to your state's health insurance commissioner and/or your state and federally elected representatives to enlist their help. Inform them of your health needs and what has occurred with your health plan insurance claims. Notify your insurance company that you have requested help from your state's health insurance commissioner and other agency representatives to resolve difficulties meeting your health care needs.

You can make a difference! Remember the expression, "the squeaky wheel gets the grease." The more you make your needs known, the more likely you will get those needs met.

Working with Insurance Providers After a Diagnosis

Once you have determined your preferred treatment with your doctor(s), find out which procedures require you to pay a co-payment and co-insurance, and how much that will be. If you buy your own insurance rather than receiving it as a benefit of employment or your spouse's employment, make sure you pay your premiums on time.

Tip: Request a case manager to speak with each time you call your insurance company.

Tip: Make notes about each call. Record the date, the name(s) of who you spoke with, and any instructions you were given. You can save and organize your records with file folders or by scanning and saving them on your computer.

If your doctor wants to refer you to one or more specialists, make sure that the specialists are covered in your plan's network. If they are not and you still want to see them, consider that you will likely be responsible for their entire fee.

Organize your records, including bills, claims, payments, records of phone calls to and from doctors and your insurance company, and letters to and from your employers, doctors, and insurance company. Include dates, who you spoke to, and a brief note of what transpired for each occurrence.

If you're required to submit bills to your insurance company, try to send them in as soon as you get them. Keep the original bills and send copies. If you're recovering from treatment, ask a loved one or a friend to help you.

Handling Claims

Keep detailed records of all the claims you submit. Note when they were submitted, whether they're still pending, and when they were paid. Also, keep copies of all paperwork related to your treatment, diagnosis, and insurance claims, including:

- Requests for sick leave
- Receipts
- Letters to and from your doctor, employer, and insurance company
- Bills from providers
- Summaries of phone calls to your insurance company, including the date, time, and person's name to whom you spoke.

Managing the Costs of Care

Learn whether the procedure you want requires you to pay a co-payment and co-insurance, and how much that will be. Ask how you are required to pay. Does your insurance company make the first payment and you are billed for the balance? Or do you pay the entire bill and then get reimbursed? If you're required to submit bills to your insurance company, try to send them as soon as you receive them. If you're recovering from treatment, ask a loved one or friend to help you. Section 13 of this *Guide* is devoted to helping you reduce and manage your health care costs.

Fighting Insurance Denials

Many insurance companies deny claims just because they know there is a good chance the consumer will not appeal. When you advocate for yourself, you let the insurance company know that you are not going to go away without a fight. Sometimes just being polite and persistent is enough to get your denial reversed.

So, how do you know if your claim is denied? An explanation of benefits (EOB), which is sent to you by your insurance company, is one way to determine what the insurance paid to the provider and how much you may still owe. The EOB should also disclose if your claim was denied. If the insurance company portion of the payment shows $0, this can indicate a denial. The payment amount should be followed by a Reason Code(s). This code provides an explanation for the lack of payment. The insurance company may also send you a letter confirming the denied medical claim and detailing the reason(s) for denial.

Make sure to keep copies of all correspondence you receive from the insurance company, including denial letters, approval letters, and EOBs. Make copies of all correspondence you send to the insurance company, including letters, your health history, medical files, doctor's letters, etc. As mentioned earlier in this section, keep a written record of all phone calls with the insurance company

If your insurance company denies a claim, follow the steps below:

Tip: For no cost, the Patient Advocate Foundation will help you solve your insurance issues. Contact them by calling 1-800-532-5274, by email at help@patientadvocate.org, and on their website at www.patientadvocate.org.

Step 1. Check Your Plan

Make sure the benefit you want is included. Make a note of the part of the policy that leads you to believe your claim should not have been denied.

Step 2. Organize Your Records

Collect and organize all information pertaining to the denied claim. Make sure you have the original bill, your EOB, any letters from the insurance company, and your insurance card before you call.

Step 3. Missing Information

Call the number provided on the letter from your insurance company; if you did not receive a letter call the customer service number. There is the possibility the claim was denied simply because of missing information. Once the missing information is provided, the claim can be reprocessed, and you may be done.

Step 4. Miscoding

Sometimes claims are denied because of miscoding. If that is the case, ask your doctor to review the coding and resubmit a request with more specific medical justification for the procedure and you may be done.

Step 5. Other Reasons for Denials

If your claim was not denied for missing information or miscoding, find out why it was denied and how you can file an appeal.

Step 6. Ask for Help

Ask the insurance provider's representative for suggestions or guidelines for appealing a denial. If you would like an appeal form, ask the insurance provider to send one via regular mail or email. If the provider doesn't have one, use the template in Addendum 2 of this *Guide*.

Step 7. Understand Your Insurance Denial Appeals Process

Make sure you have the address for the appropriate department to return the completed appeal documents.

Step 8. Keep Accurate Records

Always keep a record of the date, time, and name of the insurance company representative you talked with, along with a brief summary of the discussion. Keep this with copies of any documents you send to the insurance company.

Step 9. Get Documentation

In appealing the denied claim, you should have the opportunity to review the information the insurance company used to make its decision.

Step 10. Get Help from Your Doctor(s)

If necessary, get your doctor involved. Their office should have staff that can help explain why the procedure or care is medically necessary.

Step 11. Writing Your Appeal

Get help wording your appeal so that it mentions your medical problem and does not include words that automatically trigger denials. Talk to the person who handles insurance claims at your doctor's office. This person may be able to help you with the appeal process and provide any documentation your insurance company requires.

Step 12. Follow All Instructions

Remember each insurance company has its own appeal process. Before submitting your information, make sure you have completed and included all of the required paperwork. Once all of the documents are complete, make a copy of everything for your reference.

Step 13. When Appeals Are Denied

If your insurance company denies your appeal, in most cases you can contact them to request an external appeal. Usually this will be conducted by a medical professional or group of medical professionals who are not associated with the insurance company.

Step 14. Take Legal Action

Sometimes it takes the threat of a lawsuit to get your insurance company to approve your claim.

Send all of your correspondence to the insurance company via certified mail with return receipt. Be persistent. Remember that a denial is not necessarily the final word. Ask your insurance company to reconsider its decision, and follow up to make sure it is taking action.

Medicare[23]

Medicare is health insurance offered by the federal government to people who are 65 or older, and meet specific eligibility requirements. The specific requirements can be found on the Medicare website at www.medicare.gov. Some people qualify for both Medicare and Medicaid. This is called "dual eligibility."

Tip: Medicare coverage can be confusing. Fortunately, you can find out if your test, item, or service is covered through a feature found on the home page of the Medicare website at www.medicare.gov.

Original Medicare is a fee-for-service plan that covers many health care services and certain drugs. Usually, you can go to any doctor or hospital that accepts Medicare. With all of the recent and expected changes to Medicare, it is important for you to contact your local Medicare office to discuss your situation every time you expect to need services. At the end of your conversation you want to know as best you can what expenses Medicare will cover and what your financial obligations will be.

Medicare has four parts:

- **Part A** helps pay for hospital bills.
- **Part B** is a supplemental insurance option that pays for physician services and supplies outside of the hospital.
- **Part C** includes private health plans that are Medicare-approved.
- **Part D** is prescription drug coverage.

Part A: Hospital Coverage—The Basics

When you sign up for Medicare, you automatically get Part A. If you or your spouse paid Medicare taxes while working, you will not have to pay a monthly premium for Part A coverage. If you paid Medicare taxes for less than 7.5 years, your premium would be about $460 per month at the time of researching this book. If you paid Medicare taxes for more than 7.5 years but less than 10 years, your premium would be about $255 per month.

Part A covers much of the cost of inpatient hospital stays, including semi-private room, food, tests, and doctor's fees. However, Medicare beneficiaries still pay a portion of their costs. Part A also covers brief stays in a skilled nursing facility if certain criteria are met. In general the criteria are:

- A preceding hospital stay of at least three days and three nights, not counting the discharge day.
- An illness or condition diagnosed during a hospital stay or was the main cause of a hospital stay.
- The patient is receiving rehabilitation, or has some other ailment that requires skilled nursing supervision.
- The care being rendered by the nursing home must be skilled.

The maximum length of stay that Medicare Part A covers in a skilled nursing facility per ailment is 100 days as of the writing of this *Guide*. The first 20 days are paid for in full by Medicare, with the remaining 80 days requiring a co-payment. If a beneficiary uses some portion of his or her Part A benefit and then goes at least 60 days without receiving facility-based skilled services, the 100-day clock is reset and that person qualifies for a new 100-day benefit period.

Medicare Part A does not pay for custodial, nonskilled, or long-term care. It does not pay for help with activities of daily living (ADLs). Examples of ADLs are personal hygiene, cooking, cleaning, bathing, etc.

Part B: Medical Coverage—The Basics

Medicare Part B is optional. It can be deferred if the beneficiary or spouse is still working. However, you must sign up for Medicare Part B if you want it. The purpose of Part B is to cover physician and medical services not covered under Part A.

If you sign up, you will pay a monthly premium and a yearly deductible. The premium may increase each January, and it is deducted from your Social Security check. You are also responsible for a 20% co-payment for the services and supplies you are approved for.

If you do not sign up for Medicare Part B when you are first eligible, you may have to pay a higher monthly premium. The additional services covered typically include:

- Doctor visits (both inpatient and outpatient) at a hospital, doctor's office, or health care facility
- Laboratory tests and x-rays
- Physical therapy or rehabilitation services
- Ambulance service
- Some home health care
- Some medically necessary medical equipment
- Physician and nursing services
- Influenza and pneumonia vaccinations

- Blood transfusions
- Renal dialysis
- Outpatient hospital procedures
- Limited ambulance transportation
- Immunosuppressive drugs for organ transplant recipients
- Chemotherapy
- Hormonal treatments
- Other outpatient medical treatments administered in a doctor's office

Tip: The actual administration of medication is covered under Part B only if it is administered by the physician during an office visit.

At the time of writing this *Guide*, Part B also helps with durable medical equipment (DME). This can include canes, walkers, wheelchairs, and mobility scooters for those with mobility impairments. Prosthetic devices such as artificial limbs and breast prostheses following a mastectomy, one pair of eyeglasses following cataract surgery, and oxygen for home use are also most often covered.

Deductibles and Co-insurance[24]

After a beneficiary meets the yearly deductible, he or she is required to pay a co-insurance of 20% of the Medicare-approved amount for all services covered by Part B. Lab services are an exception, and they are often covered at 100%. You may also be required to pay an excess charge of 15% for services rendered by nonparticipating Medicare providers.

Part C—Private Health Plans (Medicare Advantage)[25]

Medicare Part C gives consumers the option to receive their Medicare (Parts A and B) benefits through private Medicare-approved health plans. When you join this type of plan you are still in Medicare. Often called Medicare Advantage Plans, private plans often cover more services and have lower out-of-pocket costs than the Original Medicare plan.

These plans are not available in all areas. They usually include: health maintenance organizations (HMOs), preferred provider organizations (PPOs), private fee-for-service plans, Medicare Special Needs Plans, and medical Savings Account (MSA) plans (such as Medicare Advantage).

Medicare Advantage plans provide hospital and medical coverage and medically necessary services. They generally offer extra benefits, including drug coverage. For people who choose to enroll in a Medicare Advantage health plan, Medicare pays the private health plan a set amount every month for each member.

Members of these plans pay a monthly premium to cover items not covered by traditional Medicare (Parts A and B). These items may include prescription drugs, dental care, vision care, and gym or health club membership. These plans often restrict members to a network of providers they can use without having to get special permission and/or pay extra. That means you may have to see the plan's doctors and go to certain hospitals to get care if you want the plan to pay its part of the expense.

Tip: If you have a Medicare Advantage plan, you don't need supplemental insurance or a Medigap policy.

Medigap Plans—The Basics[26]

Medigap policies are standardized by the Centers for Medicare & Medicaid Services. They are sold and administered by private insurance companies. They cover some of the out-of-pocket costs from Medicare Parts A and B. Medicare beneficiaries can't have both a Medicare Advantage Plan and a Medigap Policy. Medigap policies may only be purchased by beneficiaries who are receiving benefits from Original Medicare (that is parts A and B only).

Medigap plans are not like Medicare Advantage plans that use HMOs and PPOs. Examples of expenses that are usually covered by Medigap plans include co-payments, co-insurance, and the yearly Medicare deductible. However, co-insurance is only covered after the deductible is paid unless your Medigap policy pays the deductible.

Tip: A Medigap policy can only cover one person. If you are married, both you and your spouse must buy separate policies.

There can be big differences in the costs and benefits of the various plans. Therefore, the government requires that the companies providing these plans have to clearly identify that the policy is a Medicare Supplement Insurance on the front of each policy. Remember that Medicare pays for many health care services and supplies, but it doesn't pay all of your health care costs. There are costs that you must pay, for instance, co-insurance, co-payments, and deductibles.

You might want to consider buying a Medigap policy to cover these gaps in Medicare coverage, or a Medicare Advantage policy to replace your Original Medicare plan. Some Medicare Advantage plans include prescription drug coverage. You can also add prescription drug coverage by joining a Medicare prescription drug plan.

Comparing Plans and Plan Ratings

To compare health plans and Medigap policies, go to the Medicare website at www.medicare.gov. From the home page, click on "Sign Up/Change Plans," Then click on "Find & compare doctors, hospitals, & other providers." You can also compare prescription drug plans, nursing homes, hospitals, home health agencies, and dialysis facilities from the same website.

In December 2015 the Kaiser Family Foundation published a report that provided quality ratings for Medicare Advantage organizations. The ratings were based on data from the Centers for Medicare and Medicaid Services (CMS), the Consumer Assessment of Healthcare Providers and Systems (CAHPS), the Healthcare Effectiveness Data and Information Set (HEDIS) data, and the Health Outcomes Survey (HOS). New plans did not receive ratings because data was not available. Almost 60% of the Medicare Advantage programs were rated. The rated plans represented 85% of the enrollment.[27]

The report found that:

1. Private fee-for-service plans and regional PPOs had below average ratings that were significantly lower than traditional HMOs and local PPOs.

2. Nonprofit plans had higher ratings than for-profit plans.
3. Plans with contracts that began before 2004 had higher ratings than newer plans.[28]

Part D: Prescription Drugs—The Basics

Part D is prescription drug coverage provided by private companies. Everyone with Medicare can get this coverage. There is usually a separate monthly premium for this coverage. If you decide not to enroll in a drug plan when you are first eligible, you may have to pay a penalty if you join later. Part D coverage is not standardized by Medicare. Each plan is free to choose which drugs they cover and what the coverage levels are. If plans cover drugs that are excluded from coverage by Medicare, they are not allowed to pass those costs along to Medicare.

Tip: If you are dually eligible for Medicare and Medicaid, consider that Medicaid may pay for drugs not covered in a Medicare Part D plan.

Tip: To compare prescription plans, go to the Medicare website at www.medicare.gov. From the home page, click on "Drug Coverage (Part D),"then click on "Find health & drug plans."

Medicare Prescription Drug Choices

The decision to get Medicare prescription drug coverage depends on how you intend to pay for your drugs and what Medicare coverage you have. Most people with Medicare pay for drugs and have one of the five types of Medicare coverage below:

- Original Medicare only.
- Original Medicare and a Medigap policy without drug coverage.
- Original Medicare and a Medigap policy with drug coverage.
- A Medicare Advantage plan (like an HMO or PPO) or other Medicare health plan, which already includes drug coverage and other benefits.
- Dual coverage from Medicare with Medicaid drug coverage. These people currently receive comprehensive prescription drug coverage from Medicare.

If you have specific drug needs due to a medical condition, Medicare's Formulary Drug Finder lets you enter a typical combination of drugs used by people with a certain condition to find out which plans in any particular area have formularies that cover these drugs.

Joining Medicare

Individuals receiving Medicare benefits have a lot of information to go through. If you have never enrolled in Medicare and are about to do so for the first time, you will need to answer a lot of questions to make the best decision on the best coverage for you. One of the most important tools available is a handbook put out through the federal government called *Medicare & You*. The most recent government handbook can be found at http://www.medicare.gov/publications/. Consumers can also get a free and secure assessment of their personal Medicare benefits and services at www.mymedicare.gov/.

You can join Medicare every year between November 15 and December 31. At that time you can also make changes to your existing coverage. On January 1 each year your new coverage becomes effective. You can get Medicare coverage information through your doctor, state health department, city, county, or state department on aging, senior citizen centers, or other health care and senior organizations.

Medicaid

Medicaid is a state and federal partnership that provides health coverage for selected categories of people. Its purpose is to improve the health of people who might otherwise go without medical care for themselves and their children. In most cases a state caseworker will work with you. Medicaid pays for your health care if you qualify, although there are efforts to have Medicaid recipients pay a small part of their expenses.

Medicaid is a state-administered program. Each state sets its own guidelines regarding eligibility and services and sets rules for the program. Generally, if your income is low and you meet one of the following criteria, your odds of qualifying for Medicaid are good.

- Pregnant
- Parent or guardian of minor children
- Aged
- Blind

- Disabled

There are many groups of people are covered by Medicaid. Low income is only one test for Medicaid eligibility; assets and resources are also tested against established thresholds.

Medically needy persons who would be eligible except for income or assets may become eligible for Medicaid solely because of excessive medical expenses. The rules for counting your income and resources vary from state to state and from group to group. There may also be special rules for those who live in nursing homes and for disabled children living at home.

Your child may also be eligible for Medicaid coverage if he or she is a U.S. citizen or a lawfully admitted immigrant, even if you are not. However, there is a 5-year limit that applies to lawful permanent residents. Eligibility for children is based on the child's status, not the parent's. Your income does not apply to your child in this case. If another child lives with you, he or she may get Medicaid. Apply for Medicaid for your child to find out if you can get it.

People who are eligible for Medicaid may or may not also receive cash assistance from other federal programs like the Temporary Assistance for Needy Families (TANF) and/or Supplemental Security Income (SSI) programs. You should contact your state's Medicaid office to find out if you are eligible for benefits.

For the most part, you should apply for Medicaid if your income is low and you match one of the descriptions of the eligibility groups in your state, and you or your family need health care. This will allow a qualified caseworker in your state to evaluate your situation.

Medicaid does not pay money to you; instead, it sends payments directly to your health care providers. Depending on your state's rules, you may also be asked to pay a small part of the cost (co-payment) for some medical services.

Screening Tools–Know Your Benefits

To help you determine whether you are eligible for federal, state, and local programs, you can visit the Benefits.gov website at www. benefits.gov, or visit another website called BenefitsCheckUp at www.benefitscheckup.org.

When Medicaid Eligibility Starts

Coverage may start retroactively to any of the three months prior to applying, if the applicant would have been eligible during the retroactive period. Coverage generally stops at the end of the month in which a person's circumstances change. Most states have additional "state-only" programs to provide medical assistance for specified poor persons who do not qualify for the traditional Medicaid program. No federal funds are provided for state-only programs.

Low-income Medicaid beneficiaries who would otherwise become ineligible for Medicaid due to an increase in wages or hours at a job are entitled to up to 12 months of Medicaid benefits under the Transitional Medical Assistance (TMA) program. This temporary coverage increases the likelihood that low-income people who start a job or find higher-paying work will not lose the security of health coverage because they found a job or will earn higher pay.

Working with a Medicaid Case Manager

If you are getting ready to interview or hire a professional case manager for yourself, a family member, or a loved one, here are some questions you may want to ask during the interview process:

- How long have you been a case manager?
- How many people are on your case load?
- Where do you live?
- How often do you contact your client and their families?
- How do you communicate with service providers?
- Do you develop a care plan for your clients?
- How often do you review and update your clients care plan?
- What is the best way to contact you?
- What should we do in an emergency and we can't reach you?

Medicaid Planning

There are a few things you can do using Medicaid planning to rearrange your finances and legally shelter your assets from the state. The strategies can be very complicated so you may want to consult an elder law attorney to help you with the specifics. You can find qualified elder law attorneys in your area by visiting the National Academy of Elder Law Attorneys (NAELA) website at www.naela.org.

Medicaid planning helps shelter and preserve assets for heirs and provide resources for the healthy spouse. The total value of your countable assets including your income determines whether you are eligible for Medicaid. Under federal guidelines, each state has a list of exempt assets. This list usually includes items like your home, prepaid burials, term life insurance, and an automobile(s).

You can rearrange your finances so that countable assets are exchanged for exempt assets and thus are inaccessible by the state. For example, you can exchange spending your savings on nursing home bills for:

- Paying off the mortgage on you family's home.
- Prepaying for burial arrangements.
- Making home improvements.
- Purchasing one car for your healthy spouse.

Preserving assets for your children and heirs allows you to provide financial help for your loved ones. An irrevocable trust can help you accomplish this. Consult an experienced attorney about how to set this up for your circumstances because "irrevocable" means that you can't come back and change it later, or decide to end it. Also, laws vary from state to state and from year to year, so the assistance of an elder law attorney is crucial.

Property placed in an irrevocable trust will be excluded from your financial picture for Medicaid purposes. Anything that you place into the trust can be sheltered from the state and preserved for your loved ones. More often than not, the trust must be in place and funded over a specific period of time for it to be an effective Medicaid planning tool. You might be able to use an annuity to guarantee that your spouse has enough money to live on if you have to go to a nursing home.

When the state is considering a married person's eligibility for Medicaid, the couple's assets are pooled together. Your healthy spouse is generally given a resources allowance that amounts to one-half of the assets. As you can imagine this may not be much money over the long term, especially if your spouse needs to take time off from work.

If you're married, an annuity can help protect your healthy spouse. An important loophole in the current law is that your healthy spouse can use jointly owned countable assets to buy a single premium immediate annuity for his or her benefit. By doing so, you effectively convert countable assets into an income stream. Each spouse is then entitled to keep all of his or her own income instead of pooling assets. The end result is that the institutionalized spouse can more easily qualify for Medicaid.

Medicaid Planning Risks

Since laws vary from state to state and from year to year, Medicaid planning is more effective in some states and at certain times than others. For example, when you are applying for Medicaid, the state has the right to look back at your finances for a certain period of months before the application date. Generally, there is a 36-month look-back period for transfers of countable assets, along with a 60-month look-back period for similar transfers into irrevocable trusts.

Countable asset transfers for less than fair market value made during the look-back period will commonly result in a waiting period before you can start to collect Medicaid. For example, transferring your house to your children a year before entering a nursing home may make you ineligible for Medicaid for quite some time.

Without question, you should consult with an elder law attorney who is experienced at Medicaid planning in your state. He or she will be aware of the look-back periods, estate recoveries, disqualifications for Medicaid in your state, and all of the details you need to be aware of.

SECTION 5

Free and Low-Cost Health Services

If you can't afford health insurance, there are numerous other sources of free and discounted health care. Those sources include the government, free clinics, rural and community health clinics, hospitals, federal programs, Medicaid, the Children's Health Insurance Plan, pharmaceutical companies, health organizations like the American Red Cross, and charities. This section will help you find the right options for you.

Government Assistance Programs

To find government assistance programs go to https://www.benefits.gov/benefits/benefit-finder#benefits&qc=cat_1. The online screening tool is free, easy-to-use, and confidential. You do not have to include any personally identifiable information like your name, phone number, or social security number. You will be prompted to input your location and some information about your circumstances. You will answer a series of questions about yourself and get a list of government benefits programs you may be eligible for, along with information about how to apply.

Free Clinics

There are many free clinics throughout the United States that will provide services for people who do not have insurance or the income to get care from private practices. You can find a free clinic by searching on the National Association of Free and Charitable Clinics website at www.nafcclinics.org.

Rural Health Clinics

There are more than 3,500 rural health clinics (RHCs) located in rural areas throughout the United States. The purpose of a RHC is to provide primary care services in underserved rural areas. Each clinic typically provides physician services and onsite laboratory testing. However, services vary from clinic to clinic. You need to research the services of the clinic you are going to visit. Most RHCs also have arrangements with hospitals that furnish services not available at the RHC. Patients who visit a RHC may see a physician, nurse practitioner, or physician assistant. Sometimes RHCs offer home visits by a registered professional to the homebound.

You can find a list of clinics near you at http://www.wheretofindcare.com/How-to-Pick-a-Rural-Health-Center.aspx. You can search by zip code, provider name, or other more detailed information. The website also offers quality ratings based on feedback from user surveys taken by people experienced with rural health care.

Community Health Centers

The U.S. Department of Health and Human Services (HHS) provides assistance through federally funded community, migrant, and other health centers. You pay what you can afford based on your income level. Health centers are in most cities and in many rural areas. You can find the one closest to you by going to www.findahealthcenter.hrsa.gov, typing your zip code or city and state into the search box on the home page, and clicking the search button.

Health center services typically include:

- Checkups when you're sick.
- Treatment when you're sick.
- Complete care when you're pregnant.
- Immunizations and checkups for your children.
- Dental care and prescription drugs for your family.
- Mental health and substance abuse care if needed.

Local Hospitals

Do not overlook your local hospital as a source of low-cost health care. If you owe medical bills or need care, contact the department of social or patient services at the hospital where you were treated or intend to be treated. Explain your situation and ask what help they can provide.

One of the best-kept secrets is that most large hospitals have clinic systems that provide some sort of discounted care to people without insurance or free care to Medicaid patients. Many of the large hospital clinics must accept Medicaid outpatients, and in fact get paid quite well for treating them. These clinics are often staffed by skilled medical residents in training. The resident doctors have an attending physician in the clinic to consult with as needed. What's more, some of the hospitals even supply discounted medications to clinic patients.

The downside to using a large hospital clinic system is that your clinic doctor is not likely to be the one taking care of you when you are admitted to the hospital. Instead, you will be admitted as a service case, and other residents in training there will care for you. But if you chose a top-notch hospital, you could end up with better care than if you paid thousands of dollars out-of-pocket for care in a mediocre community hospital.

Clinics may be crowded, and it may be a bit more difficult to get special tests or consultations, then again, the care could end up being quite good. Also, since residencies only last a few years, you won't have the same doctor for more than three years.

Federal Programs

You can access free and low-cost care at many hospitals, nursing homes, and health care facilities throughout the country through a program called the Hill-Burton Act (HBA). Facilities that provide care through HBA are required to do so because they have received funding from the federal government. You must qualify for the discounted care by applying at the facility where you are treated. Qualification is based on your ability to afford care taking into account your income, family size, and other factors.

Hill-Burton facilities may use different eligibility standards and procedures. HBA facilities must post a sign in their admissions office, business office, and emergency room that says: "NOTICE–Medical Care for Those Who Cannot Afford to Pay," and they must provide you with a written "individual notice," called the Hill-Burton Individual Notice, that lists:

1. The types of services eligible for HBA free or reduced-cost care.
2. What income level qualifies for free or reduced-cost care.
3. How long the facility may take in determining an applicant's eligibility.

Only facility costs are covered, not your private doctors' bills. Facilities may require you to provide documentation that verifies your eligibility, such as proof of income. Although HBA facilities must provide a specific amount of free or reduced-cost care each year, they can stop once they have provided the amount specified.

You are eligible to apply for HBA free care if your income is at or below the current Department of Health and

Human Services poverty guidelines. You may be eligible for HBA care if your income is as much as two times (triple for nursing home care) the Health and Human Services poverty guidelines. Care at a HBA -obligated facility is not automatically free or reduced-cost. You must apply and be found eligible.

Tip: You may apply before or after you receive care. You may even apply after a bill has been sent to a collection agency.

Obligated facilities publish an Allocation Plan in the local newspaper each year. The Allocation Plan includes the income criteria and the types and amount of services it intends to provide at no cost or low cost for the year. When you apply for Hill-Burton care, the obligated facility must provide you with a written notice that tells you what free or reduced-cost care services you will get, or why you have been denied.

To apply for Hill-Burton free or reduced-cost care, follow the steps below:

- Find an updated list of the Hill-Burton obligated facility nearest you at https://www.benefits.gov/benefits/benefit-finder#benefits&qc=cat_1.
- Once you find a facility, contact the facility admissions or business office and ask for a copy of the Hill-Burton Individual Notice. The Individual Notice will tell you what income level makes you eligible for free or reduced-cost care, what services might be covered, and exactly where in the facility to apply.

- Go to the office listed in the Individual Notice and say you want to apply for Hill-Burton free or reduced-cost care. You may need to fill out a form.
- Gather any required documents (such as a pay stub to prove income eligibility) and take or send them to the obligated facility.
- If you are asked to apply for Medicaid, Medicare, or some other financial assistance program, you must do so.
- When you return the completed application, ask for a Determination of Eligibility. Check the Individual Notice to see how much time the facility has before it must tell you whether or not you will receive free or reduced-cost care.

The top reasons that a facility may deny your request are:

- Your income is more than the income specified in the Allocation Plan.
- The facility has given out its required amount of free care as specified in its Allocation Plan.
- The services you requested or received are not covered in the facility's Allocation Plan.
- The services you requested or received are to be paid by a governmental program such as Medicare, Medicaid, or insurance.
- The facility asked you to apply for Medicare, Medicaid, or other governmental program, and you did not.
- You did not give the facility proof of your income, such as a pay stub.

You may file a complaint with the U.S. Department of Health and Human Services if you believe you have been unfairly denied. Your complaint must be in writing and simply state the facts and dates concerning the complaint. You may call your local legal aid services for help in filing a complaint. Send your complaint to:

Director, Division of Facilities Compliance and Recovery
5600 Fishers Lane, Room 10-105
Rockville, MD 20857

Free and Low-Cost Care for Children

The federal government and states offer health insurance coverage for children through both Medicaid (up to age 21) and the Children's Health Insurance Program (up to age 19), also referred to as CHIP. These programs typically cover doctor visits, dental care, prescription medicines, and immunizations, as well as services like hospitalizations and care for children with special health care needs. The programs serve families who are not able to afford health insurance coverage in the private market or do not have coverage available to them. There may be premiums or other costs associated with this coverage, but the programs are designed to be affordable.

Medicaid[29]

You apply for Medicaid through the state you live in. Each state has different rules about Medicaid eligibility and services. For example, there are special rules for those who live in nursing homes and for disabled children living at home. If you or someone in your family needs health care, you should apply for Medicaid even if you aren't sure if you qualify, and let a caseworker in your state evaluate your situation.

Medicaid does not pay money to you. It sends payments directly to your health care providers. Depending on your state's rules, you may also be asked to pay a co-payment for some medical services. If you can't afford to pay for medical care, Medicaid can make it possible for you to get the care that you need.

Medicaid does not provide medical assistance for all poor people. Low income is only one test for Medicaid eligibility. It is available only to certain low-income individuals and to families who fit into an eligibility group that is recognized by federal and state law. Even within the eligibility group certain requirements must be met. Requirements may include your age; whether you are pregnant, disabled, or blind; your income and resources (such as bank accounts, real property, or other items that can be sold for cash); and whether you are a U.S. citizen or a lawfully admitted immigrant.

Assets and resources are also tested against established thresholds. Medically needy persons who would be eligible except for income or other assets may become eligible for Medicaid solely because of excessive medical expenses.

Medicaid coverage is also available in every state for children living below the federal poverty level. This was $20,090 for a family of three in 2016. Children up to age 21 are eligible. In addition, states must provide Medicaid coverage for children up to age 6 with incomes below 133% of the federal poverty level. This was $26,812 for a family of three in 2016. The Medicaid program served more than 25 million children in 2016.

People in Household	2016 Federal Poverty Level
1	$11,880
2	$16,020
3	$20,160
4	$24,300
5	$28,440
6	$32,580
7	$36,730

Medicaid pays for a full set of services for children, including preventive care, screening and treatment of health conditions, physician and hospital visits, and vision and dental care. In most cases, these services are provided at little to no cost to the family. Remember that Medicaid eligibility is different in most states. Also, note that poverty guidelines are different in Alaska and Hawaii.

Children's Health Insurance Program[30]

There are two ways to apply for the Children's Health Insurance program (CHIP). Call 1-800-318-2596, or fill out an application at the health insurance marketplace website at https://www.healthcare.gov/get-coverage/, or via state applications at http://www.insurekidsnow.gov/state/index.html. Just click on the state where you live and follow the instructions to apply.

Every state's program is unique, with individual eligibility rules and benefits. In general, children in families with incomes up to $44,500 per year (for a family of four) are likely to be eligible for coverage. If you don't qualify for Medicaid or CHIP, you can still get low-cost health care for your children at community health centers. The amount you pay is based on your income. You can locate community health centers in your area at http://findahealthcenter.hrsa.gov/index.html

Other Sources

Shriners Hospitals for Children is an international health care system of 22 hospitals dedicated to improving the lives of children. They provide specialty pediatric care, innovative research, and outstanding teaching programs. Children up to age 18 with orthopedic conditions, burns, spinal cord injuries, cancer, and cleft lip and palate are eligible for care at a Shriners Hospital. If approved, the services are provided with no financial obligation to families. You can call the toll-free patient referral line at 1-800-237-5055 to see if your child or a child you know qualifies.

The National Association of Free and Charitable Clinics provides information on 1,200 free clinics that are staffed by a volunteer workforce of doctors, nurses, therapists, pharmacists, nurse practitioners, and other health care professionals. Its website is www.nafcclinics.org.

Pharmaceutical Company Assistance Programs

Many people get their prescription medications free or low-cost through programs listed with the Partnership for

Patient Assistance (PPA). The PPA offers a single point of access to more than 475 public and private programs, including nearly 200 offered by pharmaceutical companies. There are no fees to get help from a PPA representative. Its website is www.pparx.org/. You can also call the PPA toll-free at 1-888-477-2669.

RxHope is a free program that helps people to get medications that they otherwise could not afford. The program offers to advocate for people by supplying information and help. Its website is www.rxhope.com.

RxAssist is a program that is sponsored by the pharmaceutical company AstraZeneca. The program offers a comprehensive database of pharmaceutical company patient assistance programs, as well as practical tools, news, and articles so that health care professionals and patients can find the information they need. Its website is www.rxassist.org/.

Needy Meds is a nonprofit organization with the mission of helping people who can't afford to pay for their medications. Its website is www.needymeds.org.

You can find an indexed list of pharmaceutical company prescription drug programs and other financial support at https://apatientsplace.com/financial-assistance-programs/.

Other Health Organizations

Benefits.gov and BenefitsCheckUp

If you want to know whether you qualify for Medicaid, financial assistance, and other government assistance programs at both the federal and state level, you can go to www. benefits.gov or www.benefitscheckup.org.

Benefits.gov is the official benefits website of the U.S. government, with information on over 1,000 benefit and assistance programs. BenefitsCheckUp is a service of the National Council on Aging. It includes both public and private programs for all 50 states and Washington, D.C. Programs are available to cover the expenses of prescription drugs, nutrition (including food stamps), general health care, and in-home health services. Organizations listed by Benefits.gov have helped more than 2 million people and provide almost $8 billion dollars in annual benefits.

Health Resources and Services Administration (HRSA) Information Center

The HRSA information center provides publications, resources, and referrals on health care services for low-income, uninsured individuals and those with special health care needs via a comprehensive website at www.hrsa.gov/index.html or toll-free at 1-888-Ask-HRSA (1-888-175-4772). Users will find detailed listings of facilities that provide free or reduced-cost health services, information on sites that provide comprehensive primary health care services for people living with HIV, listings of dental providers who provide care to people living with HIV, and more.

Foundation for Health Coverage Education

The Foundation for Health Coverage Education helps people find free or low-cost health coverage. Contact them by phone at 1-800-234-1317 or their website at https://coverageforall.org. Their stated mission is to simplify public and private health insurance eligibility information to help more people access coverage.

Breast Cancer Screenings

Use the toll-free numbers listed after this paragraph to find local and accredited facilities that provide free or reduced-fee mammograms.

National Cancer Institute's Cancer Information Service: 1-800-4-CANCER (1-800-422-6237)

The American Cancer Society: 1-800-ACS-2345 (1-800-227-2345)

National Alliance of Breast Cancer Organizations: 1-888-80-NBCO

Komen Breast Center Helpline: 1-877-GO- KOMEN (1-877-465-6636)

Breast Cancer Network of Strength: 1-800-221-2141; Spanish Hotline: 1-800-986-9505

Millions of people qualify for free or low-cost health and dental coverage. In addition to the resources listed in this section there are many disease-specific charities and organizations that provide support and/or financial assistance for people struggling to access and pay for health care.

[1] Research Now. (2015). Are mobile medical apps good for our health? A new study by Research Now reveals that doctors and patients say yes. *Research Now News*. Accessible at https://www.researchnow.com/news-item/mobile-medical-apps-good-health-new-study-research-now-reveals-doctors-patients-say-yes-infographic/.

[2] Ibid.

[3] Gregg, H. (2014). A glimpse in Banner Health's telemedicine success. *Becker's Hospital Review*. Accessible at https://www.beckershospitalreview.com/healthcare-information-technology/a-glimpse-into-banner-health-s-telemedicine-success.html.

[4] Ibid.

[5] Ibid.

[6] McCains, V. (2016). Johns Hopkins study suggests medical errors are third-leading cause of death in U.S. HUB, Johns Hopkins University. Accessible at https://hub.jhu.edu/2016/05/03/medical-errors-third-leading-cause-of-death/.

[7] Fitch, A. (2014). How to spot 8 common medical billing errors. Nerdwallet blog. Accessible at https://www.nerdwallet.com/blog/health/common-medical-billing-errors/.

[8] National Committee for Quality Assurance (NCQA). (2016). The essential guide to health care quality. Accessible at https://www.ncqa.org/Portals/0/Publications/Resource%20Library/NCQA_Primer_web.pdf.

[9] Schiff, G. D., Kim, S., Abrams, R., et al. (2015). Diagnosing Diagnosis Errors: Lessons from a Multi-institutional Collaborative Project. Advances in Patient Safety, Vol. 2, pp. 255–278. Accessible at https://www.ahrq.gov/downloads/pub/advances/vol2/Schiff.pdf.

[10] Renter, E. (2015). 6 Ways to Be Your Own Health Advocate. *U.S. News & World Report*, February 2, 2015. Accessible at http://health.usnews.com/health-news/patient-advice/articles/2015/02/02/6-ways-to-be-your-own-health-advocate.

[11] American Heart Association (AHA) (2016). Why high blood pressure is a "silent killer." Retrieved from AHA website at http://www.heart.org/HEARTORG/Conditions/HighBloodPre ssure/SymptomsDiagnosisMonitoringofHighBloodPressure/Sy mptoms-Diagnosis-Monitoring-of-High-Blood-Pressure_UCM_002053_Article.jsp?gclid=CLSVudqNxdECF QwyaQode84IIQ#.WHvrWIWcGUk.

[12] Centers for Disease Control and Prevention (CDC) (2015). Healthy weight. Retrieved from CDC website at https://www.cdc.gov/healthyweight/assessing/bmi/adult_bmi.

[13] American Heart Association (AHA) (2016). What your cholesterol levels mean. Retrieved from AHA website at http://www.heart.org/HEARTORG/Conditions/Cholesterol/Ab outCholesterol/What-Your-Cholesterol-Levels-Mean_UCM_305562_Article.jsp#.WHvuC4WcGUk.

[14] Ibid.

[15] Ibid.

[16] U.S. Preventive Services Task Force, Screening for Colorectal Cancer: U.S. Preventive Services Task Force Recommendation Statement. AHRQ Publication 08-05124-EF-3, Oct. 2008. Agency for Healthcare Research and Quality, Rockville, MD. Accessible at https://www.uspreventiveservicestaskforce.org/Page/Documen t/UpdateSummaryFinal/colorectal-cancer-screening.

[17] American Cancer Society (ACS) (2016). Skin cancer prevention and early detection. Retrieved from http://www.cancer.org/cancer/skincancer-melanoma/moreinformation/skincancerpreventionandearlydete ction/index.

[18] National Institute of Mental Health (NIH) (2016). Men and depression. Retrieved from NIH website at https://www.nimh.nih.gov/health/publications/men-and-depression/index.shtml.

[19] Semigran, H.L., J.A. Linder, C. Gigengil, and A. Mehrotra (2015). Evaluation of symptom checkers for self-diagnosis

and triage: audit study. *British Medical Journal* http://dx.doi.org/10.1136/bmj.h3480.

[20] Kubler-Ross, E. (1969). *On Death and Dying*. New York: Macmillan.

[21] DeBronhart, D. (2015). NLM director Donald Lindberg is retiring. Speak up: What's next for the library. E-Patient Dave blog. Retrieved from http://e-patients.net/archives/2015/02/nlm-director-donald-lindberg-is-retiring-speak-up-whats-next-for-the-library.html.

[22] Firger, J. (2014). 12 million Americans misdiagnosed each year. CBS News. Accessible at http://www.cbsnews.com/news/12-million-americans-misdiagnosed-each-year-study-says.

[23] CMS. (2017). "Medicar.e" Centers for Medicare & Medicaid Service website. Accessible at https://www.cms.gov/Medicare/Medicare.html.

[24] CMS. (2017). "Medicare 2017 costs at a glance." Centers for Medicare & Medicaid website. Accessible at https://www.medicare.gov/your-medicare-costs/costs-at-a-glance/costs-at-glance.html.

[25] CMS. (2017). "Medicare Advantage Plans." Centers for Medicare & Medicaid website. Accessible at https://www.medicare.gov/sign-up-change-plans/medicare-health-plans/medicare-advantage-plans/medicare-advantage-plans.html.

[26] CMS. (2017). "How to compare Medigap policies." Centers for Medicare & Medicaid website. Accessible at https://www.medicare.gov/supplement-other-insurance/compare-medigap/compare-medigap.html.

[27] Jacobson, G., Gold, M, Damico, A, Neuman, T., and Casillas, G. (2015). Medicare Advantage 2016 Data Spotlight: Overview of Plan Changes. The Henry J. Kaiser Family Foundation website. Accessible at http://kff.org/report-section/medicare-advantage-2016-data-spotlight-overview-of-plan-changes-quality-ratings.

[28] Ibid.

[29] CMS. (2017). 2017 Program Requirements. Centers for Medicare & Medicaid Services website. Accessible at https://www.cms.gov/Regulations-and-Guidance/Legislation/EHRIncentivePrograms/2017ProgramRequirements.html.

[30] CMS. (2017). Centers for Medicare & Medicaid Services (CMS): Children's Health Insurance Program (CHIP). Centers for Medicare & Medicaid website. Accessible at https://www.hhs.gov/about/budget/fy2017/budget-in-brief/cms/chip/index.html.

www.ingramcontent.com/pod-product-compliance
Lightning Source LLC
Chambersburg PA
CBHW060505280326
41933CB00014B/2875